Antipsychotics for Non-psychotic Disorders

A Sample Mental Health Dissertation

N.I. Nwokolo

ISBN-13: 978-1541296749
ISBN-10: 1541296745

For my beloved Daddy and Mummy, without whose unrelenting encouragement this would not have been possible.

With many thanks to God, my tutors and lecturers, and all my teachers through the years.
I am grateful.

Abstract

Atypical or second-generation antipsychotics (SGAs), originally introduced for schizophrenia, have increasingly in recent years been prescribed off-label, gaining attention for their side-effects and costliness. This project aims to review current best practice guidance to identify common non-psychotic psychiatric disorders in which sound evidence has been found for the use of atypical antipsychotics, and to use this information in producing a local prescribing guideline chart for use in an NHS psychiatric service.

A pilot study was carried out in preparation for a clinical audit to examine relevant baseline prescribing practice in the community mental health teams (CMHTs) comprising the local psychiatric service. Subjects were adult outpatients who had attended a psychiatric clinic in one CMHT over the course of a year, and had been prescribed an atypical antipsychotic for a non-psychotic psychiatric disorder. 75% were found to have a primary diagnosis of borderline personality disorder, 20% of depression, and 5% of post-traumatic stress disorder. The most commonly-prescribed antipsychotic was Aripiprazole.

From literature searches, six relevant research studies, systematic reviews of randomised controlled trials, were selected for critical appraisal. Based on their findings, as well as NICE guidelines, a draft prescribing guideline was drawn up, tabulating atypical antipsychotics recommended for adjunctive use in common non-psychotic psychiatric disorders. Plans for dissemination of the research information, audit findings and guideline in the psychiatric service have been outlined, as well as strategies for evaluating potential outcomes of this proposed organisational change.

Contents

Antipsychotics for Non-Psychotic Disorders; A Sample Mental Health Dissertation

Abbreviations

APA – American Psychiatric Association

BCPFT – Black Country Partnership NHS Foundation Trust (UK)

BPD – Borderline personality disorder

CASP – Critical Appraisal Skills Programme

C.I. – Confidence interval

CMHT – Community mental health team

DSM – Diagnostic and Statistical Manual of Mental Disorders

EBP – Evidence-based practice

EPS – Extrapyramidal side-effects

FDA – Food and Drug Administration (U.S.)

GAD – Generalised anxiety disorder

GP – General Practitioner

ICD-10 – International Classification of Diseases

MDD – Major depressive disorder

NHS – National Health Service

NICE – National Institute for Health and Care Excellence

OCD – Obsessive-compulsive disorder

O.R. – Odds ratio

PPI – Patient and Public Involvement

PTSD – Post-traumatic stress disorder

RCTs – Randomised controlled trials

SGAs – Second-generation antipsychotics

SNFT – Salisbury NHS Foundation Trust (UK)

SSRIs – Selective serotonin reuptake inhibitors

List of Figures
Page

List of Tables

Chapter 1: Introduction and Background

The term 'antipsychotic' refers to the group of medications used to control symptoms of psychosis and reduce psychomotor excitement. The earliest, chlorpromazine, was introduced in 1952, and along with others such as haloperidol, is described as a 'first-generation' antipsychotic (Cowen et al, 2012). Atypical or second-generation antipsychotics (SGAs), such as risperidone, olanzapine, quetiapine and aripiprazole, were progressively introduced from 1993, initially for schizophrenia. Widely considered more tolerable than first-generation antipsychotics, they have increasingly been prescribed off-label for several non-psychotic psychiatric disorders, and are now among the most commonly-prescribed medications worldwide (Crystal et al, 2009, McKean and Monasterio, 2014).

Non-psychotic disorders in which SGAs have been used include depression (Maher et al 2011, Spielmans et al 2013), anxiety (Depping et al 2010), post-traumatic stress disorder (Ipser and Stein 2012), obsessive-compulsive disorder (Veale et al, 2014), borderline personality disorder (Stoffers et al, 2010) and even insomnia (Maher et al 2011). Marston et al (2014) found, in a UK primary care study of antipsychotic prescriptions, that over 50% were issued for patients with no record of psychosis. The commonest indications for antipsychotic prescriptions were anxiety, depression and insomnia, although national guidelines such as those by NICE only supported their use in psychotic or treatment-resistant depression (NICE 2012), obsessive-compulsive disorder (NICE 2005b) and borderline personality disorder (NICE 2009).

Over the last two decades, SGAs have largely replaced first-generation antipsychotics, which are now rarely used, and SGAs have in recent years gained attention for concerns about their safety, costliness, and increasingly prevalent use, including widespread off-label prescribing (Alexander et al, 2011). Antipsychotics are believed to exert their antipsychotic action by binding to, and blocking, dopamine receptors in the brain (Depping et al 2010), particularly the D_2 subtype. Their additional affinities for various other neurotransmitter receptors such as the serotonergic, histaminergic and adrenergic, can produce antidepressant, sedative and anxiolytic effects (Cowen et al 2012), which are often helpful and form the basis for their use in a variety of psychiatric disorders.

SGAs differ significantly in their pharmacological properties, but fall into two main groups, selective D_2-receptor antagonists such as sulpiride and amisulpiride, which are substituted benzamides highly selective of the D_2-receptor, and $5\text{-}HT_2\text{-}D_2$-receptor antagonists such as risperidone, olanzapine, quetiapine and aripiprazole, which act on $5\text{-}HT_2$ (serotonin) receptors in addition to dopamine receptors, and have varying effects on other receptors such as anticholinergic, histaminic and adrenergic (Cowen et al 2012).

The four most commonly-prescribed atypical antipsychotics at the time of writing are risperidone, olanzapine, quetiapine and aripiprazole (Alexander et al 2011). Risperidone is a potent antagonist at both $5\text{-}HT_2$ and D_2 receptors, and also has alpha-adrenoreceptor-blocking properties, causing mild sedation and hypotension. Olanzapine is a slightly weaker D_2 receptor antagonist, and also has anticholinergic and histamine H_1-receptor-blocking activity, giving it strong sedative effects. Quetiapine has modest $5\text{-}HT_2$ receptor antagonism and even weaker D_2 receptor antagonism, and shows very low propensity to cause movement disorders. Aripiprazole is a partial dopamine agonist with $5\text{-}HT_2$ receptor-blocking and $5\text{-}HT_{1A}$ agonist properties. It is activating, and can cause dopaminergic side-effects like insomnia, nausea and vomiting. It is less likely to cause weight gain or significant extrapyramidal side-effects (Cowen et al 2012).

Although most SGAs carry lower risk of extrapyramidal side-effects (neurological symptoms including movement disorders, stiffness and tremors) than first-generation antipsychotics, over time they have to varying extents been linked with significant metabolic and cardiovascular side-effects including weight gain, hyperglycaemia, precipitation of diabetes mellitus, raised serum lipids, increased prolactin levels and cardiac arrhythmias (Kendall, 2011, Maher et al, 2011, Cowen et al 2012, Spielmans and Parry 2010, Spielmans et al, 2013, Semple and Smyth 2013). It is therefore crucial that their use is always clearly indicated.

Spielmans and Parry (2010) indicate that marketing tactics by major drug companies, including suppressing negative research findings on efficacy and side-effects, and exaggerating positive ones, mean that publicly available evidence on antipsychotics may not represent with full accuracy the data underlying these medications. The paper also highlights the practice of 'disease-mongering' (expanding diagnostic paradigms of psychiatric disorders beyond their usual criteria) to achieve more sales.

Alexander et al (2011) found that in 2007 the four leading SGAs; quetiapine, aripiprazole, olanzapine and risperidone, each had US sales exceeding $1 billion, and they estimated the cost of off-label SGA use in the US in 2008 at $6 billion. They also found that the cost of an atypical prescription increased by 43% between 2004 and 2008, and 54% of off-label SGA prescribing in 2008 was described as 'off-label use with uncertain evidence.' According to Kendall (2011), in 2003 the cost of antipsychotics in the USA equalled the cost of paying all their psychiatrists. SGAs in that year alone were found to achieve sales of $7.5 billion (Leucht et al, 2009).

Ilyas and Moncrieff (2012) examined trends in prescribing and costs of psychotropic medications in England between 1998 and 2010, using data from the Prescription Cost Analysis, which details the number and net cost of NHS community prescriptions. They discovered rising trends in prescription of psychotropic medications including antipsychotics, and that antipsychotics had overtaken antidepressants as the costliest psychotropics. They found that numbers of antipsychotic prescriptions issued increased by 5.1% each year. Costs of antipsychotics increased by 22% each year, in total a 286.4% increase over 13 years examined. In 2010 alone, 7,575 500 community prescriptions (not including hospital or private ones) were issued for antipsychotics, with a net cost of £281,814 100.

I work as a career-grade psychiatrist in a multidisciplinary community mental health team (CMHT), supervised by a consultant psychiatrist. The CMHT has a senior nurse team manager, and also employs community psychiatric nurses, psychologists and a support worker. Figure 1 is an organisational flowchart outlining its structure.

Our patients are mostly those with psychoses such as schizophrenia and bipolar disorder, but also include many with debilitating non-psychotic disorders such as depression, anxiety, obsessive-compulsive disorder, personality disorders and post-traumatic stress disorder. Many have psychiatric comorbidities (more than one psychiatric disorder occurring together in one individual).

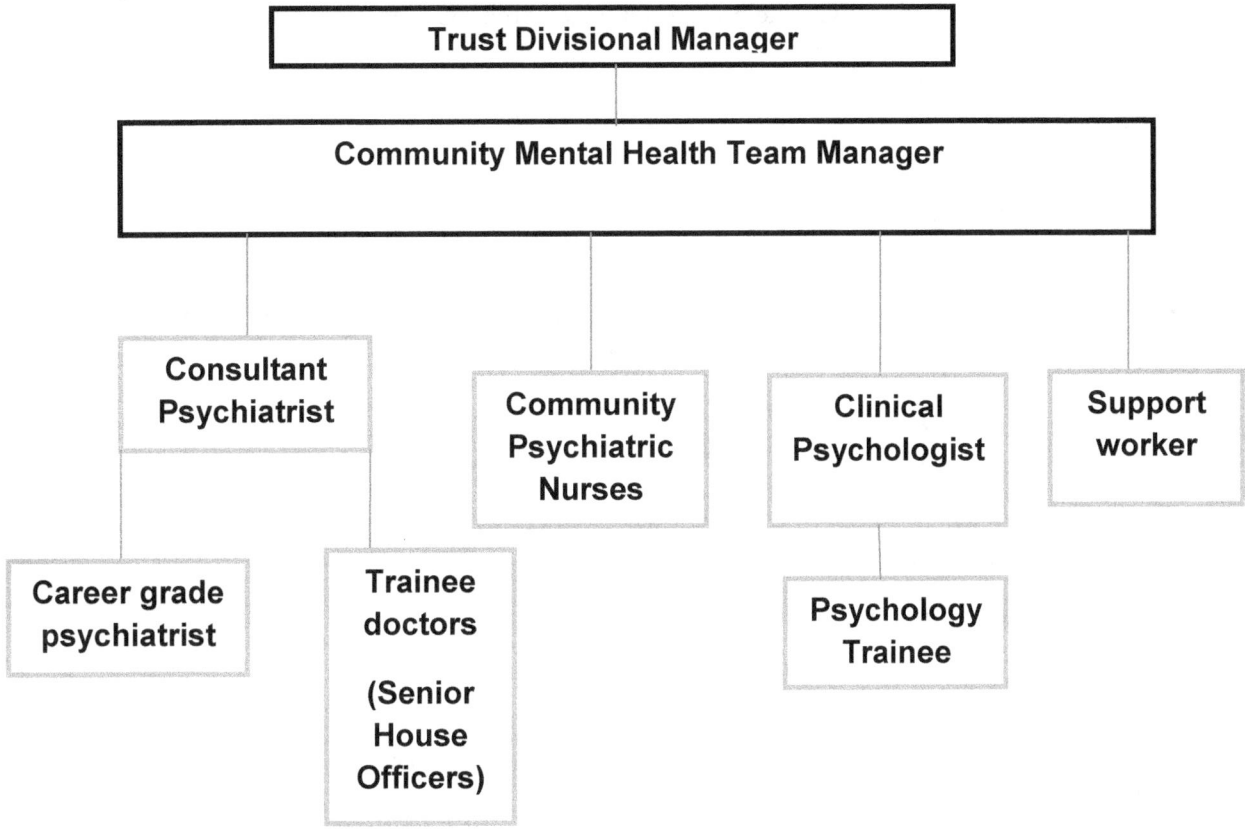

Figure 1. Organisational flowchart of community mental health team

My role frequently involves prescribing SGAs, and this project's first objective was to review current best practice guidance to identify the common non-psychotic psychiatric disorders in which a sound evidence base has actually been found for the use of SGAs, in adults aged between 18 and 65. Literature searches were carried out, with the selection and critical appraisal of a number of relevant studies, and based on the information sourced a draft prescribing guideline was drawn up.

The project's second objective is to use the research evidence towards encouraging best prescribing practice in the local CMHTs. A pilot study was carried out in 'CMHT X,' one of the community mental health teams, in preparation for a full-scale clinical audit examining baseline SGA prescribing for non-psychotic disorders in the service's six CMHTs. Strategies were drawn up for the dissemination of audit findings and the guideline, as well as for evaluation of potential outcomes of the dissemination.

EBP question:

An important early step in evidence-based practice is defining one's subject area of interest in terms of a clinical question that needs answering; this focuses searches for evidence (Aveyard and Sharp, 2013). The 'PICO' acronym, displayed in Table 1, was devised to help healthcare researchers in framing evidence-based clinical questions, highlighting patient population (P), intervention (I), comparison (C), and outcome (O) of interest as components. 'T' is sometimes added, for time frame, but is not always relevant. PICO helps in finding research evidence to answer questions by identifying key words for database searches and clinical outcomes to evaluate (Fineout-Overholt and Johnston 2005, Wallace, 2011, Aveyard and Sharp, 2013, Biggam, 2015).

Table 1. **Using PICO in defining my EBP question**

Population	Adult patients with non-psychotic psychiatric disorders treated with atypical antipsychotics
Intervention	Treatment with atypical antipsychotics
Comparison	Adult patients with non-psychotic psychiatric disorders not treated with atypical antipsychotics
Outcome	Improvement in psychiatric symptoms

Using the PICO framework, this is the clinical question that will be addressed:

In which non-psychotic psychiatric disorders have atypical antipsychotics been found effective?

The benefit of the PICO method is that it enables researchers concentrate on components central to their research, making it easier to locate relevant studies (Biggam, 2015). It provides an efficient framework for searching electronic databases and retrieving only articles relevant to the clinical question (Melnyk et al 2010). PICO components may have different meanings depending on whether quantitative or qualitative research is being considered (Aveyard and Sharp 2013).

As a result of the evidence-based information acquired in the course of this project, I hope a few colleagues and I will be better placed to select effective SGAs for non-psychotic psychiatric disorders, and that patients will benefit.

Chapter 2: Evidence-gathering and management of the evidence

Selecting key words from the EBP question is the first step in searching for evidence (Fineout-Overholt and Johnston 2005). Used individually and then combined, key words and phrases identified by the PICO framework help retrieve relevant articles from research databases by setting limits to narrow down results (Melnyk et al 2010). Inclusion and exclusion criteria also need to be decided on, for example date limiters, searches in English only, and so on.

Databases like Google are not specific enough for health-related information; a subject-specific search engine or database such as MEDLINE or CINAHL is needed. These contain references for clinical topics, and produce search results in form of academic journal articles allocated indexed key words stored by the database. When a key word is entered, the database produces a list of references of papers it holds which have been allocated that word (Aveyard and Sharp 2013).

The key words used in my database searches were:

Atypical antipsychotics, non-psychotic, depression, second-generation, second-generation antipsychotics, off-label, OCD, pharmacotherapy, post-traumatic stress disorder, systematic review.

Wallace (2011) recommends the Cochrane Library as the best start for clinical database searching; it offers high-quality, independent clinical evidence and rigorous systematic reviews (Fineout-Overholt et al, 2008, Aveyard and Sharp 2013, Biggam 2015). PubMed Central is the free, full-text version of MEDLINE, the most widely-searched health database, and is user-friendly (Wallace 2011, Greenhalgh 2014).

The Cochrane Library was visited first in my searches, and using the 'advanced search' facility, limiters restricted the search to recent articles, published between 2009 and 2016. The term 'atypical antipsychotics' identified the intervention of interest. The first search came up with 35 articles out of a possible 9511. With the same limiters, the search term 'atypical antipsychotics AND non-psychotic' was then tried, an attempt to incorporate patient population (P) in addition to intervention (I). The Boolean term 'AND' normally reduces the number of results in a database, as both terms entered have to be present in the article for it to be recognised by the database (Aveyard and Sharp 2013). This particular search resulted in no articles.

Individual psychiatric diagnoses were then tried as the population parameter, and 'atypical antipsychotics AND depression' was entered. This yielded seven results, but none was suitable. Using the same limiters, 'second-generation antipsychotics' was entered as an alternative term for atypical antipsychotics. This yielded 27 articles. Two were selected (Depping et al 2010 and Stoffers et al 2010), on use of SGAs in anxiety disorders and borderline personality disorder respectively.

PubMed Central was now visited, and the term 'atypical antipsychotics off-label' was entered, this time limiting the search to the last 5 years. There were 405 results. 'Second-generation off-label' produced 1020 results. Again, an individual diagnosis was tried as well, and 'second-generation off-label OCD' was entered, for obsessive-compulsive disorder. This yielded 25 results, and two relevant articles were chosen (Marston et al 2014, Veale et al 2014). The term 'systematic review antipsychotic off-label depression' was tried on PubMed Central with the same limiters, and produced 390 results. On the first page, a paper on adjunctive treatment of depression with SGAs (Spielmans et al 2013) was available, and was also selected.

The third database was Google Scholar, a personal favourite. It is free, and provides links to PDFs when full-text articles are available. It does not have much scope for filtering searches (Greenhalgh 2014), so returns vast numbers of results. 'Atypical antipsychotics AND off-label AND systematic review' was entered, with date limiters of 2010 to 2016. 3990 results came up, but fortunately the first paper listed was a systematic review on off-label use of atypical antipsychotics (Maher et al 2011). There were two more useful papers also on the first page (Alexander et al 2011, Crystal et al 2009).

Again on Google Scholar, with the same date limiters, was entered: 'pharmacotherapy AND post-traumatic stress disorder AND systematic review.' 9280 results came back, but near the top of the page was Ipser and Stein (2012), a systematic review on SGAs in post-traumatic stress disorder. By this time there was a sufficient number of articles for critical appraisal, so the search was concluded.

As displayed in Table 2, some searches were more successful than others in retrieving small numbers of results. The Cochrane Library was particularly good in this respect, probably because it is limited to systematic reviews (Wallace 2011). Google Scholar produced large numbers of articles despite use of the Boolean character 'AND,' but fortunately relevant articles were found on the first pages of both searches. Greenhalgh (2014) notes that this pattern of searching, while not perfect, is common among clinicians.

Table 2. Summary of the searches

Database	Key words	Limiters	Search results	Articles retrieved
Cochrane Library	'atypical antipsychotics'	2009-2016	35	0
Cochrane Library	'atypical antipsychotics AND non-psychotic'	2009-2016	0	0
Cochrane Library	'atypical antipsychotics AND depression'	2009-2016	7	0
Cochrane Library	'second-generation antipsychotics'	2009-2016	27	2 (Depping et al 2010, Stoffers et al 2010)
PubMed Central	'atypical antipsychotics off-label'	2011-2016	405	0
PubMed Central	'second-generation off-label'	2011-2016	1020	0
PubMed Central	'second-generation off-label OCD'	2011-2016	25	2 (Marston et al 2014, Veale et al 2014).

PubMed Central	'systematic review antipsychotic off-label depression'	2011-2016	390	1 (Spielmans et al 2013).
Google Scholar	'atypical antipsychotics AND off-label AND systematic review'	2010-2016	3990	3 (Maher et al 2011, Alexander et al 2011, Crystal et al 2009).
Google Scholar	'Pharmacotherapy AND post-traumatic stress disorder AND systematic review'	2010-2016	6540	1 (Ipser and Stein 2012).

Presenting information in tables summarises data, makes it more easily understandable, and enables important comparisons (Provenzale and Stanley 2006). Data from six of the selected articles were entered into the Sadler-Moore deconstruction tool; a completed sample is in Appendix 1. As indicated, the tool is designed to help with identifying the stages of a study's research process prior to critical review. It also helps in assessing the comparative quality (hence validity) of each research study, allowing side-by-side comparisons of individual aspects of each study with those of others.

The articles selected for critical appraisal are quantitative studies, and are all systematic reviews of randomised controlled trials (RCTs); these are considered the most scientifically rigorous study design (Crowe and Sheppard 2011, Ipser and Stein, 2014, Biggam, 2015).

Systematic reviews are highly valued from both academic and policy viewpoints; they are not only limited to using data from randomised controlled trials (Crowe and Sheppard 2011), but RCTs are considered the 'gold standard' research design for evaluating treatment outcomes (Sackett, 1996). In the traditional hierarchy of evidence for assessing effectiveness of interventions, RCTs are level 2, surpassed only by systematic reviews of RCTs, which are seen as level 1, the strongest evidence for clinical decision-making (Melnyk and Fineout-Overholt 2005, Greenhalgh 2014).

There are different hierarchies of clinical evidence depending on the kind of research study being considered, but for studies considering treatment interventions the hierarchy in Table 3 is traditionally used (Aveyard and Sharp 2013). The forms of evidence are listed in descending order of importance.

Table 3. Hierarchy of clinical evidence for treatment interventions (Aveyard and Sharp 2013)

1.	Systematic reviews and meta-analyses
2.	Randomised controlled trials (RCTs)
3.	Cohort studies, case controlled studies
4.	Surveys
5.	Case reports
6.	Qualitative studies
7.	Expert opinion
8.	Anecdotal opinion

Tables 4a and b are data extraction tables used alongside the Sadler-Moore deconstruction tool, and summarise the findings of the systematic reviews.

Table 4a. Data extraction from the systematic reviews

Authors	Aim	Design	Study population	Sample size
Depping et al (2010)	Evaluating efficacy and tolerability of second-generation antipsychotics as monotherapy or adjuncts in anxiety disorders.	Quantitative; systematic review	People with GAD, panic disorder and phobias.	4144
Spielmans et al (2013)	Systematic review of efficacy and safety profiles of second-generation antipsychotics as adjuncts in depression.	Quantitative; systematic review and meta-analysis	People with current MDD and inadequate response to at least one course of antidepressants.	Not given; 14 RCTs.
Maher et al (2011)	Systematic review of efficacy and safety of second-generation antipsychotics in off-label psychiatric conditions.	Quantitative; systematic review and meta-analysis	Patients treated with atypical antipsychotics for off-label psychiatric disorders	Not given; 393 trials or studies.
Veale et al (2014)	Systematic review and meta-analysis on clinical effectiveness of atypical antipsychotics augmenting an SSRI in OCD.	Quantitative; systematic review and meta-analysis	Adults with OCD unresponsive to at least one trial of an SSRI or clomipramine.	493 participants; 14 studies.
Ipser and Stein (2014)	Review of RCTs and systematic meta-analysis on the efficacy of pharmacotherapy for PTSD.	Quantitative; Review and systematic meta-analysis	Adults diagnosed with PTSD treated with pharmacotherapy.	Not given; 37 studies.
Stoffers et al (2010)	To assess the effects of drug treatments in patients with borderline (emotionally unstable) personality disorder.	Quantitative; systematic review of RCTs	Adult patients with a formal diagnosis of borderline personality disorder.	1742 participants; 28 trials.

Table 4b. Data extraction from the systematic reviews (continued)

Authors	Data collection	Summary of findings	Hierarchy of evidence
Depping et al (2010)	Cochrane controlled trial registers and clinical trials.gov searched. 11RCTs included, comparing 3 atypical antipsychotics with placebo, benzodiazepines, pregabalin or antidepressants. Two authors extracted data independently.	GAD responded significantly better to quetiapine than placebo, but weight gain, EPS, sedation or drop-out due to side-effects more likely. Olanzapine added to antidepressants significantly reduced anxiety, but produced significantly more sedation and weight gain. No difference found with risperidone.	1
Spielmans et al (2013)	4 databases searched, with APA new research abstracts, drug manufacturers' clinical trial registries and other unpublished studies. 14 RCTs included, comparing 4 adjunctive antipsychotics to placebo for treatment-resistant depression.	All 4 second-generation antipsychotics studied (aripiprazole, quetiapine, risperidone and olanzapine+fluoxetine combination) showed statistically significant effects on remission of depression, but several adverse side-effects such as akathisia, weight gain, sedation and metabolic problems were seen.	1
Maher et al (2011)	6 databases searched for RCTs in English comparing 8 atypical antipsychotics with placebo, other atypicals, or other medication for adult off-label conditions. Independent article review and study quality assessment undertaken by 2 investigators.	Evidence was demonstrated only for a few off-label conditions treated with atypicals. Quetiapine showed significant benefit in GAD, and risperidone in OCD. Aripiprazole, olanzapine and risperidone showed small benefit for behavioural symptoms in dementia, but adverse events likely with olanzapine and risperidone. Increased risk of strokes and death in the elderly. Evidence did not support use of Second-generation antipsychotics in substance misuse, eating disorders or insomnia. Adverse side-effects common.	1

Veale et al (2014)	4 clinical databases, international clinical trial registries and pharmaceutical databases searched for RCTs comparing the effects of atypical antipsychotics with placebo for adults with OCD. Manufacturers were contacted about unpublished data. No publication date or publication status restrictions. At least 2 authors reviewed studies for inclusion.	Two studies found Aripiprazole effective in OCD in the short-term. There was a small effect size for risperidone or antipsychotics in general in the short-term. They found no evidence for the effectiveness of quetiapine or olanzapine in comparison to placebo.	1
Ipser and Stein (2014)	5 clinical databases searched for placebo-controlled RCTs of pharmacotherapy for adults diagnosed with PTSD.	Risperidone resulted in significant symptom severity in PTSD after 8 to 10 weeks. Adjunctive olanzapine significantly reduced symptom severity and sleep disturbance after 8 weeks. Significant weight gain was noted. Some positive results on PTSD symptom severity were also seen with SSRIs, venlafaxine, mirtazapine and impiramine (antidepressants), as well as lamotrigine (mood stabiliser).	1
Stoffers et al (2010)	Bibliographic databases searched, reference lists of articles followed up, reearchers in the field contacted. Two authors selected trials, assessed quality and extracted data independently.	Findings were suggestive in supporting the use of second-generation antipsychotics in borderline personality disorder, as well as mood stabilisers and omega-3 fatty acids, but most effect estimates were based on single studies. Total BPD severity was not significantly influenced by any medication.	1

These tables provided a helpful framework for critical appraisal, the next stage of the project. Critical appraisal of research studies is a key component of carrying out systematic reviews (Crowe and Sheppard 2011), and its purpose is to assess a study's relevance, strengths and limitations, with a view to determining how helpful its evidence is in answering the research question (Aveyard and Sharp 2013).

To assist critical appraisal of the six studies, I used the CASP (Critical Appraisal Skills Programme) checklist for systematic reviews as a framework (CASP 2013). A CASP table drawn up for the Maher et al (2011) study is in Appendix 2. Appraisal tools help to provide a systematic and rigorous approach to reviewing research papers (Aveyard and Sharp 2013). The CASP appraisal tool has 10 screening questions distributed under 3 initial question/subheadings, which deal in turn with the validity of a review's findings, its results, and its applicability to local patients. The CASP tool provides 'hints' under each question to provide a little more in-depth guidance to critical appraisal, but Aveyard and Sharp (2013) caution that it does not provide an exhaustive list of aspects to consider. I also referred to guidance on critical appraisal and reviewing research manuscripts by Provenzale and Stanley (2006), Aveyard and Sharp (2013) and Greenhalgh (2014).

Crowe and Sheppard (2011) found that many peer-reviewed critical appraisal tools lacked rigour in their design, and few were designed to assess the quality of research. Some were not being validated or reliability tested themselves. The authors identified 22 items, listed in 8 categories, which are generally included in critical appraisal tools. Among these, the CASP tool covered study objectives, research design, results and external validity. In systematic reviews, sampling is already dealt with in the individual primary studies chosen.

Chapter 3: Critical appraisal of the evidence

Issues affecting validity

The validity of a study means the level to which the research accurately measures and reports what it says it does (Aveyard and Sharp 2013).   All the selected studies are systematic reviews of RCTs, which are the highest-level primary studies to review in seeking evidence on clinical interventions (Aveyard and Sharp 2013).   Veale et al (2014) is a UK study.   Maher et al 2011, and Spielmans et al 2013 are American, while Stoffers et al (2010) and Depping et al (2010) are by Cochrane researchers in Germany.   Ipser and Stein (2014) is South African.   Researchers on all studies were affiliated to medical, psychiatric, psychological or epidemiological institutions.   Each described a clearly-focused aim.   The Cochrane studies (Stoffers et al 2010 and Depping et al 2010), in accordance with the database's high recommendation (Greenhalgh 2014) were impressively detailed, with in-depth descriptions of their methodology.

Database searches for RCTs were thorough in all reviews, notably Stoffers et al (2010), who had no language restrictions and tried to identify all relevant published and unpublished evidence. Spielmans et al (2013) included unpublished data and publications in other languages to reduce the risk of publication bias, but were unable to obtain data from three authors of relevant studies, and excluded one small risperidone trial because they could not extract its data.   Depping et al (2010) used published RCTs. They identified RCTs for only 3 SGAs, and no trials on panic disorder or specific phobias.   Maher et al (2011) only included studies published in English, and found no studies on off-label use for 3 SGAs.

All studies were thorough in assessing study quality; a number documented that two or more of their authors had selected trials and extracted data independently (Stoffers et al, 2010, Depping et al 2010).   Risk of bias was addressed in all studies.   Depping et al (2010) noted incomplete or selective outcome reporting in some trials, while Spielmans et al (2013) felt blinding may have been compromised by antipsychotic side-effects.   Maher et al (2011) and Depping et al (2010) observed that many trials they included had been sponsored by pharmaceutical companies, possibly introducing positive publication bias.   One writer of Ipser and Stein (2012) had received research grants and/or consultancy honoraria from several pharmaceutical companies, and their meta-analysis included open-label studies that did not control for placebo effect.

Some study limitations were identified by the authors which could affect study validity (CASP 2013).   These included: small number of studies and possible publication bias (Ipser and Stein 2014), unidentified, unpublished or excluded studies (Maher et al 2011), short duration of antidepressant use in one study and selective data publication (Veale et al 2014), lack of reporting of adverse events with the antipsychotics (Spielmans et al 2013, Stoffers et al 2010), limited data on two antipsychotics Depping et al 2010) and small sample sizes in individual studies (Stoffers et al 2010).

The studies were carried out in different countries, but were mostly consistent in confirming high rates of known adverse physical side-effects with SGAs (Depping et al 2010, Spielmans et al 2013, Ipser and Stein 2014, Veale et al 2014), including sedation, weight gain, extrapyramidal side-effects, altered glucose metabolism, hyperlipidaemia and hyperprolactinaemia.   None appeared to address specifically the risk of cardiac QT prolongation on ECG with antipsychotics, but this may be because clinical trials tend to be short-term, usually lasting weeks rather than months (Veale et al 2014). Maher et al (2011) highlighted the increased risk of thromboembolism, observing that higher rates of mortality and sudden cardiac death had been found even in the non-elderly.

Findings related to psychiatric disorders

Below is a discussion of findings of the systematic reviews in relation to psychiatric disorders. Relevant recommendations of NICE (the National Institute for Health and Clinical Excellence) are also included. NICE is an independent organisation which provides national health guidance in the UK and publishes clinical guidelines and quality standards on various disorders (BCPFT 2015, NICE 2002, 2005a &b, 2007, 2009, 2011, 2012, 2015). Its guidelines are frequently used as the basis for standards in clinical audits (Potter et al, 2010).

In some cases, NICE recommendations differed somewhat from those suggested by the systematic reviews, but with a number of the disorders the systematic reviews took place some years after the publication dates of the latest available NICE guidelines.

Depression (ICD-10 code F33)

Depression, a very common psychiatric disorder, has a prevalence of 5 to 10% in primary care, and possibly as high as 30% in the general population; depressive disorders are the fourth cause of disability worldwide (Semple and Smyth 2013). Depression can be mild, moderate or severe, and its main symptoms include persistent low mood, loss of interest and enjoyment, and reduced energy. Numerous other symptoms including disturbed concentration, sleep and appetite, suicidality and even psychotic symptoms can be present (WHO 1992). This project only deals with non-psychotic depression.

Recommended initial treatment of depression is with psychological interventions such as cognitive behavioural therapy (CBT), and if indicated selective serotonin reuptake inhibitor (SSRI) antidepressants (NICE 2012). Only when psychological interventions and trials of different antidepressants have failed does NICE (2012) recommend possibly augmenting antidepressant therapy with an antipsychotic such as aripiprazole, olanzapine, quetiapine or risperidone.

Depping et al (2010) found that depression responded significantly better to quetiapine than placebo. Their results suggested that quetiapine monotherapy was as effective in treating depression as SSRI antidepressants, but antidepressant doses used in the included trials were relatively low, which could affect validity. No difference was found with risperidone or olanzapine, but their evidence on these was limited.

Spielmans et al (2013) found statistically significant effects on remission of depression with aripiprazole, quetiapine, risperidone and a combination of olanzapine with fluoxetine, an antidepressant. Apart from risperidone, these medications were already approved by the United States FDA as adjuncts in the treatment of depression. The small-to-moderate effect sizes on depression severity measures did not differ much between antipsychotics, although the researchers noted there was limited statistical power to detect such differences because of the small number of trials available for each drug.

In 2009, Leucht et al had carried out a meta-analysis of double-blind RCTs comparing SGAs with first-generation antipsychotics, and found these SGAs significantly more effective than first generation antipsychotics in depression: amisulpiride, clozapine, olanzapine, aripiprazole and quetiapine. Risperidone was not found to be more effective. The same researchers also found that amisulpiride, clozapine, olanzapine, quetiapine, risperidone, sertindole and zotepine were associated with significantly more weight gain than haloperidol.

Spielmans et al (2013) found several problematic side-effects, including akathisia (restlessness) with aripiprazole, sedation with quetiapine, olanzapine and aripiprazole, metabolic abnormalities with quetiapine and olanzapine, and weight gain with all four medications, especially olanzapine. The researchers felt that quetiapine's sedative effect may have accounted for a substantial degree of the observed improvement in depression scores, and that results should therefore be interpreted cautiously. They noted a lack of reporting, or incomplete data, on adverse events (side-effects) in the accounts of some trials. They also cautioned that findings of effectiveness of the antipsychotics in depression needed to be weighed against abundant evidence of treatment-related harm, and benefits of treating depression with the antipsychotics were only assessed as small-to-moderate.

Generalised anxiety disorder (ICD-10 code F41.1)

Anxiety disorders are common and disabling, with a lifetime prevalence of 17% in the general population, and show high rates of treatment resistance, hence the interest in alternative pharmacological options (Depping et al 2011).

Generalised anxiety disorder (GAD) is characterised by generalised and persistent anxiety. Other symptoms commonly include tremors, muscular tension, palpitations, dizziness, sweating and epigastric discomfort (WHO 1992). Recommended treatment is initially with psychological interventions, and then if these are ineffective, or the patient prefers medication, with an SSRI antidepressant first, and then trials of other antidepressants (NICE 2011). NICE (2011) indicated that antipsychotics should not be offered for GAD in primary care. No specific antipsychotic was recommended for use in psychiatric services.

Maher et al (2011) found statistically significant benefit in GAD with quetiapine, but classified their strength of evidence as only moderate because results were inconsistent, and all the studies involved were funded by drug manufacturers (possibly introducing publication bias). Depping et al (2010) also found that GAD responded significantly better to quetiapine than placebo, but participants on quetiapine were more likely to drop out due to side-effects, to gain weight, or to suffer from sedation or extrapyramidal side-effects. They also found that olanzapine added to antidepressants significantly reduced anxiety, but produced significantly more sedation and weight gain. Risperidone did not appear to be effective in reducing anxiety as an adjunct to antidepressants.

Depping et al (2010) identified RCTs on only 3 SGAs, olanzapine, quetiapine and risperidone. Apart from weight gain, their study did not emphasise metabolic side-effects of SGAs. They identified RCTs for only 3 out of a possible 10 SGAs, and felt their evidence was incomplete. 10 of their trials were short-term, and only one long-term, which could limit external validity. All their trials were sponsored by one pharmaceutical company, and they noted that pharmaceutical companies were known to emphasize the advantages of their own products while highlighting problems with competitor compounds. They did not exclude sub-clinical forms of anxiety, thus affecting external validity; psychiatric outpatients tend to have very severe levels of anxiety. They admitted that the overall quality of their evidence was 'rather low,' as there was a high risk of bias from incomplete and selective outcome reporting.

Emotionally unstable personality disorder (ICD-10 code F60.3)

Emotionally unstable (borderline) personality disorder is estimated to have a prevalence of 1.5% in the general population (Stoffers et al 2010). It is associated with affective instability, lack of impulse control, disturbed self-image, feelings of emptiness, interpersonal relationship difficulties, recurrent self-harm and suicidality (WHO 1992). While it also frequently features symptoms present in other psychiatric disorders, such as depression, anxiety and sometimes even psychotic symptoms (Stoffers et al 2010), there is no specific medication for the disorder itself (NICE 2015).

Dialectical behaviour therapy, a psychological intervention, is the treatment of choice for patients with emotionally unstable personality disorder that self-harm (NICE 2009). NICE also outlines other important aspects of management such as risk assessment, crisis management, symptomatic treatment, and treatment of comorbid psychiatric disorders. It recommends that antipsychotics can be used for transient psychotic symptoms in borderline personality disorder, but should not be used for medium to long-term treatment, and not for the individual symptoms/behaviour associated with the disorder. NICE (2015) recommends that these patients should be prescribed antipsychotic or sedative medications only for short-term crisis management or comorbid conditions.

Stoffers et al (2010) found significant effects with aripiprazole in reducing impulsivity, anger, depression, paranoid symptoms and anxiety associated with borderline personality disorder. Patients treated with aripiprazole were also less likely to self-mutilate. With olanzapine, significant reductions in affective instability, anger, paranoia and anxiety were found, but self-damaging behaviour was more likely. Also, olanzapine participants experienced significant adverse physical effects including increased appetite, weight gain, sedation, dry mouth, increased lipids and prolactin, and altered full blood count and liver indices.

Stoffers et al (2010) admitted that most of their results were based on single study findings, and most of their study sample sizes were low, resulting in low statistical power to detect significant effects. The use of different assessment instruments by various studies also made comparability difficult. They found little data on side-effects, and strongly recommended that known adverse effects of medications be taken into account when choosing medication options. They observed that participants with comorbid psychiatric disorders should not be excluded from studies, as these were common in patients with borderline personality disorder; they felt the studies might not adequately reflect the characteristics of clinical settings with regard to patient characteristics and duration of interventions.

Obsessive-compulsive disorder (ICD-10 code F60)

The prevalence of obsessive-compulsive disorder (OCD) is 0.5 to 3% of the general population (Semple and Smyth 2013). It is characterised by recurrent obsessional thoughts (distressing ideas, images or impulses entering the individual's mind repeatedly) and compulsive acts or rituals which the individual often views as preventing some objectively unlikely harmful event. Anxiety symptoms are often present, and there is a close relationship between obsessional symptoms, especially thoughts, and depression (WHO 1992).

Recommended treatment of OCD is initially with psychological therapies, and if required, SSRI antidepressants (NICE 2005a). NICE recommends that antipsychotics can be used adjunctively to antidepressants if the condition proves resistant to initial treatment, but does not specify any particular antipsychotic. They recommend that antipsychotics should not be used as monotherapy in OCD.

Maher et al (2011) found significant benefit from risperidone in OCD, while Veale et al (2014) found limited evidence of low dose risperidone and aripiprazole in the short term, noting that aripiprazole was associated with less risk of weight gain, sedation and prolactin increase compared to other antipsychotics. Aripiprazole had a larger effect size (1.11) in treating OCD than risperidone (0.53). They admitted that most of their studies were sponsored by drug manufacturers, which could cause publication bias.

Veale et al (2014) recommended that other measures such as cognitive behavioural therapy or adding clomipramine (a tricyclic antidepressant) to an SSRI should be tried before an antipsychotic was considered, that antipsychotics should be reviewed after 4 weeks to determine efficacy, and that future studies of SSRI augmentation with aripiprazole should be followed up in the long term. They identified limitations of their review: two studies had provided incomplete data, SSRIs were used only for a short duration in some studies, and there was only a small number of studies and participants for each antipsychotic. They also cautioned that trials on off-label prescribing had been exempted from industry pledges on transparency, which increased the likelihood of selective data publication. These factors could lead to the overestimation of treatment benefits, or affect external validity.

Post-traumatic stress disorder (ICD-10 code F43)

5 to 9% of the general population develop post-traumatic stress disorder (PTSD), in which there is dysregulation of the sympathetic nervous system and hyperarousal (Ipser and Stein 2012). It arises as a delayed or protracted response to a stressful event or situation of an exceptionally threatening or catastrophic nature, and typical symptoms include reliving the trauma in intrusive memories (flashbacks), nightmares, numbness, emotional blunting, detachment, panic, hyperarousal, insomnia, aggression, avoidance of cues reminiscent of the original trauma, and commonly, anxiety and depression (WHO 1992). The risk of developing PTSD after a traumatic event is 8 to 13% for men, and 20 to 30% for women (Semple and Smyth 2013).

PTSD is frequently chronic, and associated with significant morbidity, poor quality of life, and high personal, social and economic costs. It also represents a risk factor for other mood and anxiety disorders, as well as substance misuse. It is characterised by a range of neurobiological disruptions including changes in the hypothalamic-pituitary-adrenal axis, as well as alterations in the serotonergic and noradrenergic neurotransmitter systems (Ipser and Stein (2012).

NICE (2005a) recommends initial treatment with psychological therapies such as trauma-focused cognitive behavioural therapy or eye movement desensitisation and reprocessing (EMDR), augmented with pharmacological therapy if ineffective. SSRI antidepressants are the recommended first-line pharmacotherapy, but not all patients respond (Ipser and Stein 2012). NICE (2005a) recommends a trial of different antidepressants before considering olanzapine as an adjunct if the condition still proves resistant.

Maher et al (2011) found moderate evidence of benefit for risperidone in PTSD. Ipser and Stein (2012) also found risperidone effective in reducing symptom severity in PTSD. They also found that olanzapine augmentation of an SSRI significantly reduced symptom severity and sleep disturbance, but patients gained significant amounts of weight in comparison to placebo. Limitations in their study included some smaller-sized studies, a combination of data from self-rated as well as observer-rated scales, open-label trials without controls in the meta-analysis, one author having links to 12 pharmaceutical companies (risk of publication bias), and some participants in one risperidone study taking benzodiazepines (sedatives) as well.

Panic disorder (ICD-10 code F41)
Panic disorder has a lifetime prevalence of 1.5 to 3% (Semple and Smyth 2013). Its essential features are recurrent attacks of severe anxiety which are not restricted to any particular situation, and are therefore unpredictable. Symptoms vary, but can include palpitations, chest pain, choking sensations, dizziness, feelings of unreality, and a fear of dying, losing control or going mad (WHO 1992). NICE (2011) recommends psychological treatments, followed by antidepressants. It does not recommend using antipsychotics in panic disorder, and Depping et al (2010) could not find any trials of SGAs in this condition.

Other psychiatric disorders
SGAs have also been used in dementia (Maher et al 2011), and for controlling aggression in autistic spectrum disorders and behavioural disturbances in people with learning disabilities (Semple and Smyth 2013). Caution with SGAs in the elderly has been advised in recent years due to the discovery of increased risk of strokes and mortality with these medications in this age group (Maher et al 2011). These three disorders are not frequently encountered in my own day-to-day practice, and are not included in the scope of this project.

Conclusions in regard to the EBP question:
My EBP question was, 'In which non-psychotic psychiatric disorders have atypical antipsychotics been found effective?' Systematic reviews have shown some evidence of effectiveness of SGAs as adjuncts in treating depression (Depping et al 2010, Spielmans et al 2013), generalised anxiety disorder (Maher et al, 2011, Depping et al 2010), emotionally unstable personality disorder (Stoffers et al 2010), post-traumatic stress disorder (Maher et al 2011, Ipser and Stein 2012), and obsessive-compulsive disorder (Maher et al, 2011, Veale et al 2014). SGAs are also sometimes used in dementia (Maher et al 2011), autistic spectrum disorders, and learning disabilities (Semple and Smyth 2013).

Apart from some elderly participants in the Maher et al (2011) study, the populations appeared comparable to local patients (Western adults, mostly white Caucasian, with common psychiatric disorders). The SGAs mostly featured in the studies, quetiapine, risperidone, olanzapine and aripiprazole, are readily available in the UK. Findings should therefore be relevant to local psychiatric patients, but a few issues could affect generalizability. Treatments given in the studies were for limited periods, in some cases less than 12 weeks (Depping et al 2010, Spielmans et al 2013). Most psychiatric patients take psychotropics for years (Ilyas and Moncrieff 2012), and this needs to be taken into consideration when choosing treatments. Longer-term effects will only be properly uncovered by longer clinical trials.

Additionally, many 'real-world' psychiatric patients have severe psychiatric symptomatology, suffer from more than one psychiatric disorder, and are on multiple psychotropics, all of which affect clinical response. Severely-ill patients are unlikely to be included in placebo-controlled trials, which could limit the generalizability of findings (Cowen et al 2012). Spielmans et al (2013) admitted that patients in their placebo groups might not be representative of patients in some clinical practice settings because of the inclusion and exclusion criteria of various studies.

Unfortunately, most SGAs have been found to have significant physical side-effects (Veale et al, 2014, Spielmans et al 2013, Depping et al 2010). Costs of the medications and the incompleteness of evidence supporting their use in non-psychotic disorders must also be considered (Alexander et al, 2011), and their benefits should always be weighed against risks (Haw and Stubbs, 2007, Marston et al, 2014). When prescribing antipsychotics, there needs to be monitoring of the patient's side-effects, weight, serum glucose, lipids and prolactin (NICE 2012).

Anxiety disorders (including GAD, OCD and PTSD) tend not to be as debilitating or life-threatening as psychosis or severe depression, so given the health risks of SGAs they might be best considered as a last resort, or for short-term use, in these conditions. For the same reason, it may be unadvisable to use them in treating primary insomnia. With borderline personality disorder, due to its frequent high-level emotional distress, suicidality and impulsivity, SGAs might be worth trying earlier, especially in crisis situations.

For the benefits of prescribing SGAs in non-psychotic disorders to be 'worth the harms and costs' (CASP 2013), impairment and/or distress resulting from the psychiatric condition needs to be significant, as well as unresponsive to the usual recommended interventions.

Chapter 4: Project description and implementation

This project describes the production of a local prescribing guideline based on the literature review and NICE guidelines on SGAs recommended for use in specific non-psychotic disorders.

A pilot study was carried out in 'CMHT X,' one of the community mental health teams comprising the local psychiatric service, to prepare for a full-scale clinical audit examining relevant baseline prescribing patterns in the service's six CMHT's. Pilot studies enable potential problems to be detected before the main audit (NICE, 2002). The plan is to re-audit a year after the full-scale baseline audit and guideline dissemination, to assess the guideline's effect on prescribing patterns.

This intervention should be achievable at low cost, an important consideration in financially-straitened times; service managers are likely to favour projects that are cost-effective as well as clinically effective (Potter et al, 2010). Clinical audits are also achievable in reasonably short time spans, without necessarily involving large numbers of patients (Fawkes, 2000). As with most audits, data will be collected retrospectively (NICE 2002), without live patient interviews, so confidentiality should be the only significant ethical issue. Stages of the project are described below.

Seek approval from the relevant authorities

As required by the trust, a copy of the project's audit planner (Table 6) was submitted by email, along with a copy of the data collection tool and details of the standards of care being compared against (NICE guidelines and systematic reviews). The Clinical Effectiveness facilitator confirmed registration of the audit by email, explaining that registration numbers were not currently being issued.

Clinical audits are routine NHS practice, and do not require approval from a research ethics committee (Fawkes 2000, Potter et al 2010). The trust's audit guidelines (BCPFT 2015) indicate that ethical considerations for audits include preserving patient confidentiality (all data is anonymised, omitting names of patients and clinicians), benefit to patients outweighing any risks, and no harm resulting from the process.

To obtain organisational support, an audit topic must be interesting and relevant to clinicians and trust management (Potter et al, 2010). Antipsychotic prescribing fulfils these requirements, given these medications' widespread use and costs. Audits need to be supported by the local clinical audit team, to receive advice, ensure sound methodology and increase opportunities for influencing changes in practice (Potter et al, 2010).

To publish a local guideline, approval will be needed from my line manager (consultant), team and service managers, the clinical tutor, and local corporate governance bodies such as the Medicines Management Committee and Clinical Effectiveness unit.

Pilot study prior to baseline audit

NICE (2002) defines clinical audit as 'a quality improvement process that seeks to improve patient care and outcomes through systematic review of care against explicit criteria and the implementation of change.'   In clinical audit, current practice is measured against a defined and desired standard, providing a method for reflecting on and reviewing clinical practice by evaluating how close it is to best practice (Hardman and Joughlin 1998, Tidy and Harding 2014, SNFT, 2015).   It is recognised by NHS commissioners, providers and regulators as an effective way of monitoring healthcare quality, encourages compliance with recommended clinical standards, and can improve patient outcomes (BCPFT 2015).   19th century Crimean War nurse Florence Nightingale was an early clinical audit pioneer, recording patient mortality rates and seeing them reduce with hygiene measures (Fawkes, 2000).

'Medical audit' was introduced to the NHS by the 1989 Department of Health White paper 'Working for Patients' (Department of Health 1989), formally established in the NHS in 1993 (Fawkes, 2000), and further emphasised around 1997 with the introduction of clinical governance, of which it is an integral part.   Clinical governance is the framework through which NHS organisations are accountable for continually improving the quality of their services and safeguarding high standards of care (Hardman and Joughlin 1998, Johnston et al, 2000, NICE 2002).   The term 'clinical audit' is used nowadays, as it is now multidisciplinary (Palmer, 2002).   Effective clinical audit helps demonstrate where changes are needed, although change derived from audit may be slow as it has to compete with other management agendas (Potter et al, 2010).

As in Figure 2, stages of clinical audit are generally represented as a cycle (Benjamin, 2008, Tidy and Harding, 2014).

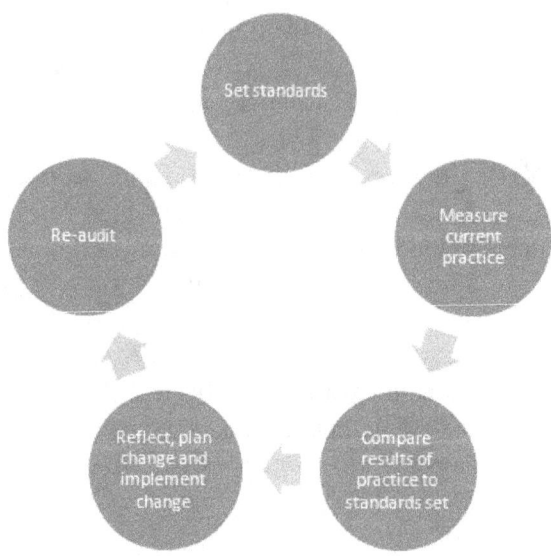

Figure 2. The Audit Cycle (Tidy and Harding, 2014)

Standards having been set by the systematic reviews and NICE guidelines, the next step was measuring current practice.

Pilot studies test audit design, data collection tools and general procedure on a small sample before the full-scale audit (Hardman and Joughlin 1998), and help to assess the feasibility of the main audit

(Potter et al, 2010). For the pilot, electronic health records were audited of patients aged between 18 and 65 who had attended an outpatient clinic at 'CMHT X' between January and December 2015, and had been prescribed SGAs for non-psychotic disorders. Data were collected retrospectively, with no live patient interviews. However, the storage and sharing of patient health records can impact on the rights and privacy of service users; legislation on the handling of medical records includes the Data Protection Act 1998 and the Freedom of Information Act 2000 (Data Protection Act 1998, Beach and Oates 2014).

BCPFT audit guidelines specify that all clinical activity must take account of the Data Protection Act 1998 and the Caldicott Principles (Caldicott 2013), and comply with the NHS Confidentiality Code of Practice (2003), which stipulates that service users are made aware that their information may be recorded, shared and used to support local clinical audit (BCPFT 2015). One major method of data protection in the trust is that access to electronic patient records is granted only to authorised staff members via use of private passwords.

To obtain the patient sample for the pilot, outpatient appointments from the psychiatric clinic were searched through for the period of one year from January 2015. There were over 500 appointments registered for the period. Referring to electronic patient records, only 21 patients seen during the course of the year had been prescribed SGAs for non-psychotic disorders. The 21st was over 65, the maximum age being considered in this project, and so was omitted from the pilot. Basic patient demographic details, antipsychotics prescribed, and primary and comorbid diagnoses were recorded on the audit tool. Patients were identified only by a serial number, with no patient-identifiable information used (Data Protection Act 1998, Potter et al 2010).

Table 5 is the audit planner designed for this project, based on models by BCPFT (2015) and Hardman and Joughlin (1998). It identifies the audit's aims and methodology, comparison standards, inclusion criteria and other relevant details of the patient sample, ethical concerns, necessary resources, project lead, team and location, and finally proposed arrangements for reporting and re-auditing.

Table 5. Clinical audit planner
(Based on models by BCFT 2015 and Hardman and Joughlin 1998).

	PROJECT DETAILS
Audit title:	'Atypical antipsychotics in non-psychotic disorders.'
Reason for audit:	To assess current (baseline) prescribing patterns of atypical antipsychotics for non-psychotic disorders in 'CMHT X'
Aims/objectives:	To determine which non-psychotic disorders atypical antipsychotics are currently being prescribed for, and which medications are being used. To encourage evidence-based prescribing of atypical antipsychotics for non-psychotic disorders in the psychiatric service.
Explain how this will benefit patient care:	Ensuring that patients get the most effective medications.

Standards/guidelines:	1. NICE guidelines on treatment of depression, generalised anxiety disorder, obsessive-compulsive disorder, post-traumatic stress disorder and borderline personality disorder. 2. Systematic reviews : Stoffers et al (2010) Depping et al (2011) Maher et al (2011) Ipser and Stein (2012) Spielmans et al (2013) Veale et al (2014).
Audit criteria:	Patients aged between 18 and 65 who attended a psychiatric clinic in 'CMHT X' between January and December 2015, and were prescribed atypical antipsychotics for non-psychotic disorders.
Sample size:	20 patient records fulfilled above audit criteria.
Audit Methodology:	Type: Retrospective Source: Electronic patient records (Care Notes).
Audit tool:	Data collection tool designed.
Patient information to be collected:	Age Sex Ethnicity Diagnosis Atypical antipsychotic prescribed
Clinical lead for project:	Name: Job title:
Proposed project team:	Names: Job titles:
Group:	Mental Health
Service area:	Community
Location	UK
Is this a re-audit?	No.
What professions are involved in this audit?	Medical.
Are any non-trust organisations involved in this audit?	No.
Service user involvement:	Indirect only; data collection is retrospective.
Resources:	Audit tool design, review of patient records and data analysis to be carried out by project lead.
Ethics/confidentiality:	In accordance with Data Protection Act and Caldicott Principles.

Date form completed:	
Proposed report date:	
Reporting arrangements:	Clinicians' academic forum.
Proposed re-audit date:	1 year following first audit report.

Table 6a is the data collection tool devised for the pilot and baseline audit. Appendix 4 contains Table 6b, the same audit tool completed with patient data from the pilot, and Table 6c, the tool slightly adjusted for the proposed re-audit.

Table 6a. Data collection tool for pilot study and baseline audit

Patient Serial no.	Age	Sex	Ethnicity	Primary diagnosis	Any psychiatric comorbidities	Atypical antipsychotic	Use supported by NICE guidelines/systematic review findings?
1							
2							
3							
4							
5							
6							
7							
8							
9							
10							

Hardman and Joughlin (1998) suggest that there is no one 'correct way' of collecting data for clinical audit, but that as with research, clinical information needs to be collected in a way that is both valid and reliable. They define 'validity' as the degree to which what is supposed to be measured is being measured, and 'reliability' as the degree to which what is desired to be measured is consistently measured. The data collection tool was designed by selecting relevant variables such as psychiatric diagnoses, antipsychotics prescribed, and relevant research evidence. Basic demographic details such as age, sex and ethnicity were also added; these could be helpful in future studies.

Arriving at psychiatric diagnoses is not always clear-cut; clinicians may disagree on diagnosis when considering the same patient. Diagnosis in routine clinics tends to be based on clinical features, without the use of standardised psychometric tools, which could also impact on the reliability of the given diagnoses.

Findings of the pilot study:
With reference to the SGAs recommended for each psychiatric condition by the systematic reviews and NICE guidelines, 85% prescribing compliance was found. However, because of the limited number of cases in the pilot (20) and the fact that only one clinic was audited, few conclusions could be drawn about local prescribing patterns for SGAs in non-psychotic disorders. Pilot study results should be cautiously interpreted when making assumptions about full-scale interventions, as effects may vary (Craig et al, 2012). National audit studies indicate that approximately 40 sets of notes are required to provide a view of the care within a healthcare setting (Potter et al 2010). Experience of the pilot suggested that the full-scale audit would be feasible, although more data collectors would be needed.

Figure 3 is a bar chart showing prescribing compliance with the systematic reviews and NICE guidance as found in the pilot.

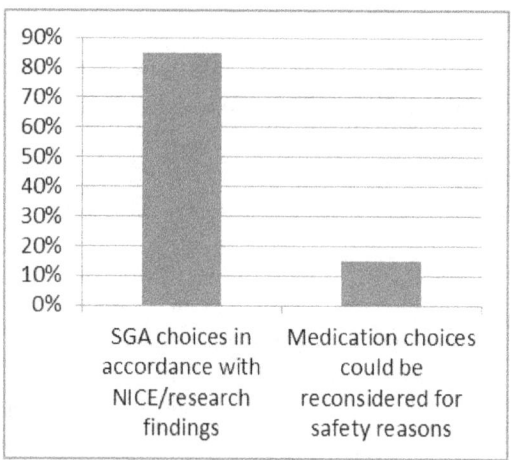

Figure 3. Bar chart showing prescribing compliance

100% prescribing compliance is an ideal standard, assuming no constraints (Benjamin, 2008) but this may not be possible or desirable, for example individual patients may not tolerate a particular antipsychotic.   An optimum lower standard such as 90 or 95% could be agreed by the implementation team (Potter et al, 2010, Tidy and Harding 2014).

Ages in the sample ranged from 20 to 54, with an average of 36.7.   80% were female, and 90% British Caucasian.   Figure 4 displays the sex distribution, and Figure 5 ethnic distribution.

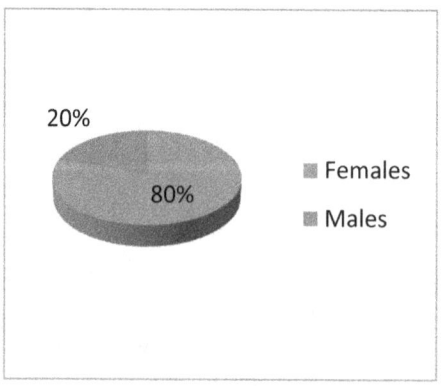

Figure 4. Sex distribution in pilot sample

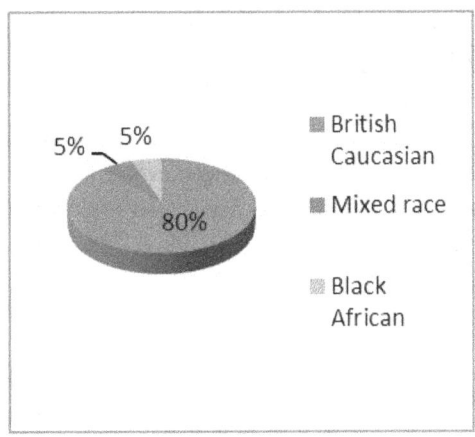

Figure 5. Ethnic distribution in pilot sample

75% had a diagnosis of emotionally unstable (borderline) personality disorder, most often diagnosed in younger females (Cowen et al 2012). 20% had a primary diagnosis of depression, and 5% had post-traumatic stress disorder. Psychiatric comorbidity is very common in mental health patients; 50% of patients with major depression also have an anxiety disorder (Cowen et al 2012). The psychiatric disorder with the most significant symptomatology was listed as the primary one, as seen in the partially-completed data collection tool in Appendix 4.

Figure 6 is a pie chart showing the distribution of primary psychiatric disorders in the sample.

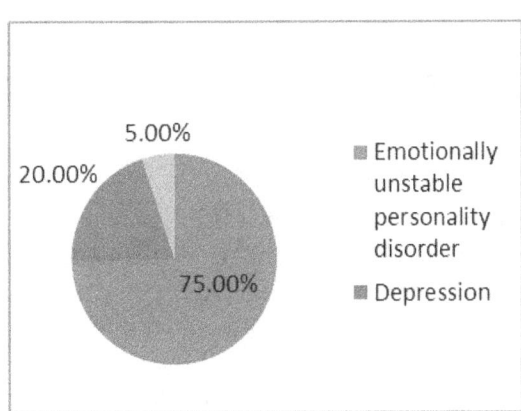

Figure 6. Distribution of psychiatric disorders in pilot sample

In 85% of cases, the SGA chosen complied with recommendations of NICE and/or the systematic reviews on the primary or comorbid diagnosis. The other 15% were cases of emotionally unstable personality disorder who had been prescribed olanzapine. Two cases of borderline personality disorder were prescribed risperidone, and one quetiapine, without depression being expressly listed as a comorbidity, but these were counted as compliant with guidelines. NICE (2015) indicates that antipsychotics can be used in borderline personality disorder for short-term crisis management or comorbidities without specifying any particular antipsychotic, and high rates of psychiatric comorbidity occur in patients with this diagnosis (Semple and Smyth 2013).

Olanzapine was found by Stoffers et al (2010) to improve some symptoms of borderline personality disorder, but was linked to increased risks of self-harm and metabolic side-effects. Ipser and Stein (2012) found significant weight gain with olanzapine. As borderline personality disorder is so often linked with depression, there could arguably be justification for any of the SGAs, but metabolic side-effects, and particularly the risk of self-harm with this group, need to be considered. For these reasons olanzapine might not be ideal.

Figure 7 shows the antipsychotics prescribed for the 20 cases. 50% had aripiprazole, 20% had risperidone, 15% had quetiapine, and 15% had olanzapine.

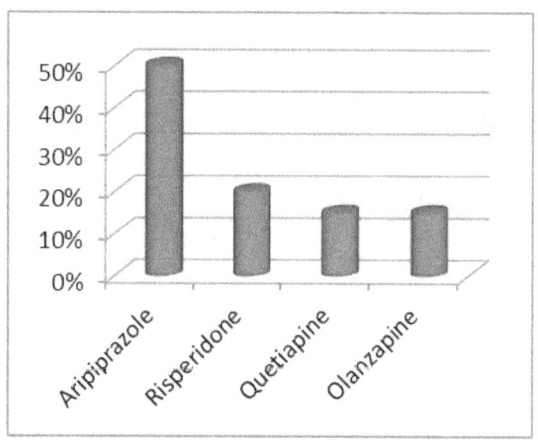

Figure 7. Antipsychotics prescribed for pilot sample

Conclusions and recommendations from pilot:

The pilot found 85% prescribing compliance with NICE guidance and/or recent systematic reviews for SGA use in non-psychotic disorders. For stronger evidence of local prescribing patterns, a full-scale baseline audit will need to be carried out, including the other CMHTs. 100% prescribing compliance may not be achievable, but 90 to 95% could be aimed for. Limitations of the pilot include small sample size, and that it was limited to one clinic, so cannot be generalised to the wider service. Also, the validity of clinical records' data is dependent on their accuracy (Potter et al 2010).

Metabolic side-effects should be taken into account when choosing SGAs. Toxicity in overdose must also be considered, especially for patients with suicidality or a tendency to self-harm. Antipsychotics in borderline personality disorder should be used on a short-term basis, for crisis management or psychiatric comorbidities.

To complete the audit cycle, an audit should be repeated after an interval of time to assess whether changes in practice have resulted in standards being met (Hardman and Joughlin 1998, Benjamin, 2008). The same procedures should be used in re-auditing, so that data are valid and comparable with the baseline audit (NICE 2002). For this project, the re-audit will take place a year after the results of the full-scale baseline audit have been presented and the prescribing guideline disseminated.

Draw up the guideline

Table 7 shows the first draft of the guideline, summarising clinical findings and prescribing recommendations from the searches and NICE guidelines. The final version will be in the format used by the trust; details will need to be obtained at that time from the Clinical Effectiveness unit.

Table 7. Draft guideline for the use of SGAs in non-psychotic disorders

Psychiatric disorder	Atypical antipsychotic recommended by NICE guidelines?	Atypical antipsychotic found effective by systematic review?
Depression	Only when treatment with antidepressants and psychological interventions have failed or shown inadequate response, consider augmenting with an antipsychotic such as **aripiprazole, olanzapine, quetiapine or risperidone** (NICE 2012).	Depping et al (2011) – significantly better response to **quetiapine** than placebo. Monotherapy with quetiapine appeared to be as efficacious as low-dose SSRIs. Spielmans et al (2013) -statistically significant effects on remission of depression with **aripiprazole, quetiapine, risperidone** and a combination of **olanzapine** with fluoxetine.
Generalised anxiety disorder (GAD)	Antipsychotics should not be offered for GAD in primary care. No specific antipsychotic recommended. (NICE 2011)	Depping et al (2011) - significantly better response to **quetiapine** in GAD than placebo. However, not officially registered for treating GAD. Maher et al (2011) - significant benefit in GAD with **quetiapine.** Depping et al (2011) - **Olanzapine** added to antidepressants significantly reduced anxiety, but produced significantly more sedation and weight gain.
Emotionally unstable personality disorder	Antipsychotics can be used to treat transient psychotic symptoms. Not for medium to long-term treatment, and not for the individual symptoms/behaviour associated with emotionally unstable personality disorder. (NICE 2009) NICE (2015) quality standards	Stoffers et al (2010) - significant effects with **aripiprazole** in reduction of impulsivity, anger, depression, paranoid symptoms and anxiety associated with the disorder. Also less likely to engage in self-mutilation.

	indicate that patients can be prescribed antipsychotic or sedative medication only for short-term crisis management or treatment of comorbid conditions.	With **olanzapine** significant reductions in affective instability, anger, paranoia and anxiety associated with the disorder. However, self-damaging behaviour more likely, and metabolic side-effects are significant.
Post-traumatic stress disorder (PTSD)	**Olanzapine** can be used as an adjunct to antidepressants and psychological interventions if condition is resistant. (NICE 2005a)	Maher et al (2011) - moderate evidence of benefit for **risperidone** in PTSD. Ipser and Stein (2012) – significant reduction of symptom severity with adjunctive **risperidone** in PTSD found. **Olanzapine** also found to significantly reduce symptom severity used as an adjunct to SSRIs. Significant weight gain with olanzapine.
Obsessive-compulsive disorder (OCD)	Antipsychotics can be used as adjuncts if condition is resistant to antidepressants and psychological interventions. Not for use as monotherapy. No specific antipsychotic identified. (NICE 2005b)	Maher et al (2011) - significant benefit from **risperidone** in OCD. Veale et al (2014) - limited evidence of low dose **risperidone** and **aripiprazole** in the short term.
Panic disorder	Antipsychotics should not be prescribed. (NICE 2011)	Depping et al (2011) - No trials identified.

Identify an EBP mentor

An EBP mentor is typically a clinician (medical or nursing) with in-depth knowledge of evidence-based practice and organisational culture change (Fineout-Overholt et al, 2011, Melnyk et al 2011). Most healthcare trusts have a clinical audit lead (Benjamin, 2008), and local audit has been found to be more effective with a committed lead clinician and management support (Potter et al, 2010). My choice for EBP mentor is the clinical tutor, the consultant psychiatrist who oversees audits and academic training. In initial discussions with the EBP mentor and CMHT manager (Gallagher-Ford et al 2011), I would present the research evidence, seek advice, arrange a multidisciplinary implementation group, agree standards (Hardman and Joughlin 1998), and plan the dissemination of information to other stakeholders.

Identify stakeholders

A committed multidisciplinary team has been found to increase the impact of clinical audit (Benjamin, 2008, Potter et al, 2010). Involving stakeholders ensures relevance (Craig et al, 2008) and new prescribing recommendations will concern prescribers, managers, pharmacists and service users (patients).

Since the 1970's, involvement of patients and the public in healthcare has been emphasised in UK health policy, and the concept of patient and public involvement (PPI) emphasises the need for citizens to have a democratic opportunity for involvement in decisions about services and healthcare quality (Department of Health 2003, Hogg 2007, Department of Health, 2008, Renedo et al, 2015, BCPFT 2015).

Raise awareness

Discussions in CMHT multidisciplinary meetings will explain the project's rationale (Gallagher-Ford et al 2011) and request feedback. Senior staff acting as unit-based 'champions' help reinforce new policies in healthcare systems (Potter et al, 2010, Melnyk et al 2011, Aveyard and Sharp 2013). The EBP mentor and CMHT nurse manager will be well placed for this role.

Appoint an implementation group

A multidisciplinary group of health professionals and patient representatives will oversee implementation of the full-scale audit, guideline and dissemination (Melnyk et al 2011, NICE 2002). Patient and carer representatives can be sourced through appropriate stakeholder organisations (BCPFT 2015), and interested trust professionals invited to join. The group will meet periodically to address aims, assess project feasibility, agree standards and audit criteria, and plan the stages of the project (Potter et al, 2010, Thornicroft and Slade, 2014).

The desired organisational change for this intervention (guideline dissemination) is for clinicians to deliberately select antipsychotics for non-psychotic disorders in line with those recommended by NICE and recent research. 'Making Informed Decisions on Change' (Cameron et al 2001) highlights a number of potential change management models and strategies relevant to the NHS. Points discussed include ensuring change management is based on sound evidence and best practice, identifying possible obstacles and facilitators (for example through a 'SWOT' analysis looking at strengths, weaknesses, opportunities and threats), and addressing concerns of managers and professionals. A formal change management approach might be considered to facilitate implementation, such as the PDSA (Plan, Do, Study, Act) cycle recommended by Potter et al (2010) and SNFT (2015).

Staff opinions can be sought by consultation in routine work meetings and by questionnaires. Aveyard and Sharp (2013) recommend that colleagues should be asked about concerns and given the opportunity to collaboratively explore solutions with the project team. Training and support might be needed to help the implementation team develop the competencies required (Nazareth 2002, NICE, 2007). An action plan for implementation of the project will be agreed, outlining changes required, assigning roles to team members, and deciding timescales (Potter et al, 2010).

Implementation of the EBP project

Advice will be sought from the trust's audit department and audit lead on procedure for the full-scale baseline audit, including ensuring the reliability and validity of instruments used. The baseline audit will then be executed. Johnston et al (2000) found that comparing one's practice with those of colleagues provided a strong impetus to changing prescribing practices. They noted, however, that some clinicians were sceptical or suspicious of audit, in some cases fearing blame, ridicule, litigation, causing offence, or considering it irrelevant, a distraction, or a form of governmental or organisational control. Confidentiality of audit findings and a 'no blame' culture is generally expected (Tidy and Harding, 2014).

Barriers to, and facilitators of, evidence-based practice, exist in health care systems (Melnyk et al 2011), and barriers can relate to individual as well as organisational factors. Individual factors include the motivation, knowledge and skills of individual practitioners, curiosity and critical thinking about best practice, while organisational factors include resources, infrastructure and leadership (Aveyard and Sharp 2013). In my trust, there is good support for audits, with an enthusiastic audit leader and supportive management. Cost concerns, colleague scepticism and potential interpersonal issues could, however, be potential barriers, although these are unlikely to prove insurmountable. Due to the modest costs anticipated, there should not be much resistance to dissemination of the guideline itself.

Organisational culture is crucial in influencing evidence-based practice; the most frequently cited barrier to successful clinical audit is lack of protected time (NICE, 2002, Benjamin, 2008). Other barriers include believing nothing can be done about a situation, lack of management interest, service cuts, and difficulties in engaging colleagues (Potter et al (2010). Greenhalgh (2014) identified reasons for clinician resistance to evidence-based guidelines: desire for clinical freedom, disagreements about evidence, defensive medicine, strategic and cost constraints, patient reluctance, infrastructure such as computer systems, lack of feedback, and confusion. Other barriers include under-staffed or overly-busy units, pressured staff, feeling threatened by change, fearing challenging established practice, feeling a lack of authority, or not seeing projects as a priority (Aveyard and Sharp 2013).

Audit presentations in my trust take place at an academic training forum; this project's pilot findings have not yet been presented. Following the full-scale baseline audit, stakeholders will be invited to a presentation (Melnyk et al 2011) of the research and audit findings. Questions and concerns will be addressed, and the guideline will be distributed and subsequently e-mailed to stakeholders. Craig et al (2008) recommend a mixture of teaching methods such as audit, feedback and reminders. Disseminating educational materials has been found to have little effect unless accompanied by selected implementation methods such as tutorials, reviews or reminders (Benjamin, 2008).

People are more open to change at certain key life stages, for example when younger, or new to a workforce (NICE 2007). As trainee doctors rotate every 4 to 6 months, the guideline could be issued to each new intake (Benjamin, 2008), and highlighted periodically at academic meetings.

Theoretical basis for the intervention:

Behaviour change is key to improving healthcare and outcomes, in regard to both healthcare workers and patients (Cane et al, 2012), and interventions for behaviour change fall into four categories, policy, education or communication, technologies and resources (NICE 2007). In this project, the desired behavioural change is that following the educational intervention (audit presentation and guideline) clinicians deliberately select antipsychotics for non-psychotic disorders in line with best practice.

Learning theories, including classical conditioning (Benson, 2007), provide a wide range of explanations for the influence of the environment on behaviour and for the development of habits, and behaviour change maintenance is promoted by a number of factors, including situating new learning in the most relevant contexts, providing retrieval cues after new learning is complete, and varying contexts in which new learning occurs (Kwasnicka et al, 2016).

Social learning theory is one of the most relevant theories for this project; knowledge and skills are acquired through social modelling, the observation and replication of other people's actions, and individuals are more likely to follow guidance from people they trust and feel connected to (Kwasnicka et al, 2016). Involving the clinical tutor and senior colleagues in disseminating the guideline should therefore encourage its use. Social learning theory also considers interactions between behaviour and its internal and external controlling conditions (Bandura and Walters, 1977). In any situation, individuals have various behavioural options, reflecting individual factors such as motivation, habits and resources, and contextual factors such as cues, opportunities and opportunity costs (Kwasnicka et al, 2016).

Cane et al (2012) validated 14 domains of theoretical constructs of behaviour containing 84 component constructs in the 'Theoretical Domains Framework' used in behavioural change and implementation research. Those likely to be of relevance here include 'procedural knowledge' (imparted to clinicians through the guideline), 'skills development,' 'practice,' 'group identity,' 'leadership,' 'organisational commitment,' 'empowerment,' 'perceived competence,' 'implementation intention,' 'outcome expectancies,' 'reinforcement' and 'distal rewards' (the expectation of positive outcomes). The authors indicated that this framework could be applied by gathering qualitative data (interviews or focus groups) or quantitative data (for example by questionnaires).

Kwasnicka et al (2016) identified five main interconnected themes representing theoretical explanations for maintenance of behavioural change: motives, self-regulation, habits, resources and contextual factors from initial behaviour change to successful maintenance. They highlighted repetition and reinforcement as key to habit formation; these can be facilitated by periodic re-auditing, repeating training sessions, and re-issuing the guideline.

Craig et al (2008) recommend that behavioural scientists be part of implementation groups, but this may not be feasible in small projects. NICE (2007) recommends that a range of behaviour change approaches should be employed, with interventions tailored to the target group. Like most health interventions, this project is a complex intervention, built from a number of interacting components (Campbell et al, 2007). It involves a number of groups of people and organisational levels, relies on a number of behaviours, and is expected to have a number of varied outcomes (Craig et al, 2012).

It is impossible to use all potentially relevant theories; one or two are typically investigated in an individual study (Francis et al, 2009). Also, no single method can be universally applied to influence all behaviour and all people, for example the unmotivated might require more information about the benefits of change than the motivated (NICE, 2007).

Chapter 5: Evaluation strategy

Evaluation is the formal assessment of the process and impact of a programme or intervention (NICE, 2007). Evaluations of health interventions are required to assess positive and negative outcomes, and to disseminate the knowledge of processes and outcomes to other practitioners (Fridrich et al, 2015). Evaluation can assess performance of practitioners, patients, healthcare systems, amenities or interpersonal processes (Donabedian, 1988), and can be relevant to clinicians, researchers, health commissioners, patients, policy-makers and the public (Craig et al, 2008). Any clinical or non-clinical service or level of care can be the subject of a service evaluation (SNFT, 2015).

Evaluation of a health intervention generally involves assessing its effectiveness and cost-effectiveness, and understanding the change process required (Craig et al, 2012). Interventions should be based on the best available evidence of feasibility, acceptability, safety, effectiveness and efficiency, and wherever possible these should be evaluated using appropriate measures (NICE, 2007).

Experimental designs are generally preferred to observational, but are not always practicable (Craig et al, 2012). Quantitative data is easier to collect and analyse (Potter et al, 2010), but a mixture of qualitative and quantitative methods is likely to be needed, for example to understand barriers to participation with an intervention (Craig et al, 2008). Qualitative data is needed to examine the experience, meaning and value of change to individuals, for example individual perspectives and interpersonal interactions (NICE, 2007, Datta and Petticrew, 2013). With non-experimental methods there should be awareness of their limitations, and findings should be interpreted with caution (Craig et al, 2012).

There are many methods of evaluating health systems, and ongoing debate about the most appropriate (Craig et al, 2012, Datta and Petticrew, 2013). Donabedian (1988), described as 'the great guru of quality measurement in healthcare' (Potter et al 2010), identified two aspects of quality, technical quality, referring to knowledge and skills of health practitioners, and interpersonal quality, the rapport between healthcare staff and patients, on which the success of technical care depends. Donabedian also believed healthcare quality could be measured in terms of structure, process and outcome (Donabedian, 1988). 'Structure' deals with how care is delivered, including facilities and staff skills. 'Process' looks at what care is delivered, while 'outcomes' deal with results.

Fridrich et al (2015) proposed a similar 'context, process and outcome' evaluation model, in which 'context' broadly includes organisational characteristics such as staffing, manager attitudes and organisational culture. 'Process' involves evaluation of the stages of the change process itself, including goals, communication, collaboration, learning, quality of intervention and participant attitudes, and 'outcome' assesses results, such as modification of attitudes and knowledge, competencies, health benefits and customer satisfaction. Good structure increases the likelihood of good process, and good process increases the likelihood of good outcomes (Donabedian, 1988).

As mentioned, this project describes a complex intervention with many interacting components (Campbell et al, 2007). For reasons of cost, resources or feasibility, it is not possible to evaluate every component; evaluators choose which to evaluate and to what extent (Fridrich et al, 2015). The main focus of this evaluation (primary outcome) will be prescribing habits following dissemination of the guideline. The re-audit a year after guideline dissemination will therefore be the main evaluation.

However, brief descriptions will be offered of methods in which other components could be evaluated if resources permitted.

This evaluation is considered with reference to the models of structure (context), process and outcome described by Donabedian (1988) and Fridrich et al (2015), and also takes guidance from other sources including the Medical Research Council Guidance (Craig et al 2008 and 2012), NICE (2002), Nazareth et al (2002), NICE (2007), Potter et al (2010) and SNFT (2015).

Setting up the evaluation:
The first step will be obtaining my line manager's approval. It is also important to ensure that the evaluation is not actually research; this could have legal implications if correct procedures are not followed, and an online 'decision tool' to clarify this prior to starting evaluation can be found at: http://www.hra-decisiontools.org.uk/research (SNFT, 2015).

Meetings will be needed with the implementation group to discuss aspects of the intervention to be evaluated and criteria on which they will be evaluated, seek advice on evaluation design from the Clinical Effectiveness office, timetable activities, identify resources and data required, assign roles, and agree timescales (SNFT 2015). Healthcare evaluations can run alongside large-scale implementation, and do not need to await the end of the project (Craig et al, 2012, Datta and Petticrew 2013).

Evaluation includes examining barriers and facilitators to implementation and change processes (Fridrich et al (2015), and considering the project's feasibility (Craig et al, 2012), including costs and impact on staff workloads (SNFT, 2015). Audits of outcome, the most relevant assessment of a patient's care, examine changes in health status of patients following treatment interventions. Assessment of patient satisfaction is increasingly important, but audit results may not necessarily represent the outcome of treatment, for example some patients may demonstrate high levels of satisfaction despite experiencing small changes in symptom control (Fawkes, 2000).

Context (structure):
The evaluation for this project has the same setting, the CMHTs of the psychiatric service. Context is the underlying frame that influences and is influenced by an intervention (Fridrich et al (2015), and complex interventions are more likely than simpler ones to depend for success on their context (Datta and Petticrew, 2013).

Implementation of healthcare interventions involves overcoming several barriers, which can include political, logistic, financial, cultural, educational and even emotional factors; organisational context has been found to be the most commonly-cited contextual barrier to implementation (Datta and Petticrew 2013). Fridrich et al (2015) feel context need not be a static, unchangeable factor; some aspects such as economic developments cannot be manipulated, but others such as manager and employee attitudes can be altered, although not easily. Some ways of evaluating context in this project include discussions with project leaders, stakeholders and managers, focus group discussions, questionnaires and documentary analysis (Fridrich et al 2015).

Organisational context can help or hinder implementation, or do both; challenges can include staffing issues such as time, resources, scepticism, difficulties with changing entrenched practices, professional support, interpersonal problems, work demands and competing priorities, or patient-related issues such as patient preferences, patient-staff interaction, recruitment and retention for trials, role of patients in managing their conditions, or from the organisation itself, such as resource shortages, leadership and organisational culture (Datta and Petticrew 2013). Any of these factors could also be facilitators, and any could be a target for evaluation.

Clinical audit can be part of evaluation, if the service is evaluated against explicit criteria (Potter et al, 2010). Audits of structure examine standards of environmental factors within which care is delivered, such as buildings, facilities, equipment, confidentiality, privacy, staff and patient records (Donabedian, 1988, Fridrich et al, 2015).

Cost considerations:
A financial analysis (SNFT, 2015) will assess the cost of delivering this intervention. In today's economic climate, NHS trusts are under pressure to reduce costs, and the trust's audit department can advise on standardised cost assessment methods (Potter et al, 2010).

Donabedian (1988) felt that to avoid inefficiency, healthcare must not be disproportionately costly compared with the health improvements produced. Including an economic evaluation makes evaluation results more useful for decision-makers, and ensures that costs of interventions are justified by potential benefits, and that appropriate outcomes are measured (Craig et al, 2008).

Process
Audits of process focus on practitioner skill and quality of clinical decisions and interventions (Fawkes, 2000). Issues considered may include training and support, communication and management structures, and how these interact with implementers' attitudes and circumstances to shape interventions (Moore et al, 2015). Evaluation can assess performance of practitioners, patients, the healthcare system, amenities and interpersonal processes (Donabedian, 1988).

The process usually assesses fidelity (whether the intervention was delivered as intended) and dose (quantity of the intervention implemented), as well as how the intervention was delivered; an intervention may have limited effects either because of weaknesses in its design or because it is not properly implemented (Moore et al, 2015). Other important considerations are causal validity, relevance to objectives of care, sensitivity and specificity of instruments and processes, timeliness and cost (Donabedian, 1988). All these will require expert guidance from the Clinical Effectiveness team.

Evaluating the clinical audits:
Audits themselves need to be monitored to improve effectiveness (Johnston et al 2000). They are evaluated as part of clinical governance; each NHS organisation is responsible for assuring the quality of clinical audit projects and programmes, and relevant frameworks and scales have been devised for trusts (NICE, 2002). Audit projects in my workplace are overseen by the Clinical Effectveness unit and clinical tutor. There is also verbal feedback received in the clinicians' academic forum.

Asking a number of data collectors to independently collect data from the same set of records, and comparing their findings, is one way of testing inter-rater reliability of data collection procedures prior to an audit (NICE, 2002).

After presentations, audit reports and recommendations are sent back to the Clinical Effectiveness unit for approval. The trust is required to produce an annual 'quality account' which includes its participation in national and local clinical audits, as well as actions taken as a consequence to improve services the trust provides (BCPFT 2015).

Evaluating training:
Following the trust's academic sessions, clinicians are asked to fill in feedback forms rating each session. These could be used in evaluation. Questionnaires (Fridrich et al 2015) could also be devised to test knowledge before and after the audit presentation and guideline dissemination.

Effectiveness of training is often difficult to measure because a wide range of variables unrelated to the training intervention can affect both training process and outcome, including individual factors such as stress, staff satisfaction and so on, which need consideration in establishing whether an outcome is due to the training intervention itself (Datta and Petticrew 2013). Nazareth et al (2002) found that educational visits by pharmacists encouraging GPs to follow prescribing guidelines were well received, and that the GPs' recall of the guidelines was good after 6 months, but there was little change in their prescribing behaviour, which was found to be constrained by other factors such as patient preferences and local hospital policy.

Evaluating stakeholder views:
Qualitative data is increasingly recognised as an essential component of health services research, and provides insight into such issues as acceptability of interventions and barriers to participation (Datta and Petticrew 2013). For this project, consultations with stakeholders will request feedback on perceptions of challenges to implementation, and examine fidelity of the intervention delivery (Moore et al, 2015). Questionnaires can be designed to assess stakeholder views before and after the project, along with reasons for objections (Fawkes 2000). For staff, views can also be sought in multidisciplinary team meetings (Melnyk et al 2011), and through group discussions and workshops (Fridrich et al 2015).

Clinical audit evaluates quality of care, which encompasses patient safety, clinical effectiveness and patient experience (Potter et al, 2010). NICE (2002) found that involving patients and good links with a patient support group could contribute to the success of an audit project. For this project, local patient groups (Potter et al 2010) will be contacted for involvement in the implementation group and for feedback. Other sources of patient opinions include direct conversations, feedback from focus groups, patients' comments or complaints, critical incident reports, and individual patient stories; the most common method of involving patients in clinical audit is satisfaction surveys (NICE 2002, Palmer 2002, Potter et al, 2010).

Patient-rated experience measures (PREMS) are questionnaires that can be used to evaluate patients' experiences of using health services, and focus on satisfaction and experience of care, while patient-rated outcome measures (PROMs) capture direct health gains (Potter et al, 2010, Thornicroft and Slade, 2014). Patients participating in the implementation group could receive PREMs designed to evaluate issues including interpersonal quality (Donabedian, 1988), such as how valued they felt as members of the team, whether their views and experiences were respected, whether they were treated in an empathic manner, and whether their confidentiality was maintained.

Evaluating the role of project lead:

As part of professional appraisal, healthcare workers in the UK periodically undergo a process of '360 degree feedback' on their work performance. Colleagues and patients provide anonymous comments via questionnaires on their impression of the professional involved. It is a means by which the professional can supplement their own self-reflection and improve performance. My role as project lead could be evaluated in a similar manner by other stakeholders in the implementation group, in addition to self-assessment.

Outcomes:

Fridrich et al (2015) defined 'outcomes' as results of the change process that are measurable and meaningful for an organisation and its stakeholders. Outcome domains include morbidity, disability, mortality, satisfaction and cost (Datta and Petticrew, 2013). The choice of outcome measures is a crucial part of evaluation design; it needs to be considered which outcomes are most important, which are secondary, and how multiple outcomes will be analysed (Craig et al, 2008). Outcomes are the ideal measure for assessing healthcare quality, but can be difficult to assess (Potter et al, 2010); many factors influence outcomes, and Donabedian (1988) states that it is not possible to know for certain the extent to which an observed outcome is attributable to a process of care.

Healthcare interventions need to be prioritised based on the best available evidence of efficacy and cost-effectiveness (NICE, 2007). Outcome evaluation generally assesses effectiveness and cost-effectiveness of an intervention, and the change process required (Craig et al, 2012). Influences of components of the intervention on effectiveness (such as leadership, intervention content, the way it is carried out, characteristics of the target population, and so on) can also be targets for evaluation (NICE, 2007).

Outcomes can be considered from the perspectives of staff, patients, carers or the public (Thornicroft and Slade. 2014). In the Nazareth et al (2002) study, the primary trial outcome was the change in prescribing practice aimed for by pharmacists encouraging GPs to comply with guidelines. Data was also collected on secondary outcomes such as number of practices agreeing to take part, number of GPs attending the programmes, and quality of information provided. Quantitative and qualitative data were collected. Modalities measured included acceptability of the message, rapport with GPs, aspects of the training that influenced GPs, barriers identified, positive and negative experiences of delivering the guidelines, and self-rated performance of the pharmacists. Methods used in data collection included group interviews, questionnaires and self-rated assessment tools.

The main focus of evaluation (primary outcome) of this project is also a change in prescribing behaviour, which will mainly be evaluated by re-audit. However, Nazareth et al (2002) forms a useful model for secondary evaluation targets in this project; resources permitting, similar secondary outcomes could also be evaluated via consultation and questionnaires for stakeholders' feedback on aspects of the process (Nazareth et al 2002, Datta and Petticrew, 2013). Feedback at similar stages of the process (raising awareness, audit presentations and stakeholder meetings) could help identify attitudinal barriers to change as well as perceptions of barriers in context and process.

The Darzi report on quality of healthcare in the UK highlighted patient experience as one of three measures of quality, along with effectiveness of care and patient safety (Darzi, 2008, Potter et al, 2010). Patient satisfaction is an important desired outcome, and patient feedback can be obtained about satisfaction with interpersonal relationships with healthcare staff, components of technical care, and outcomes of care (Donabedian, 1988). Ways of evaluating patient satisfaction used in my trust include patient feedback questionnaires, suggestion boxes and complaints.

Donabedian (1988) felt an expression of satisfaction or dissatisfaction was the patient's judgement on all aspects of care quality, but particularly concerning the interpersonal process. He suggested that no preconceived notion of successful outcomes of care precisely fits every given patient, and that all that can be hoped for is a reasonable approximation, which must be subject to individual adjustment.

Normal evaluation practice uses standardised measures (Thornicroft and Slade, 2014). However, quantitative methods may not always capture the positive impact of an intervention, so qualitative data are also used to measure patient experience (Datta and Petticrew, 2013). With standardised measures, the same outcome measures are assessed for each patient, but a particular outcome domain may not be meaningful for a particular patient. Some measures aim to address this variability, including the INSPIRE measure, in which items are selected according to patient preference (Thornicroft and Slade, 2014).

Fridrich et al (2015) classified potential outcomes of health interventions into proximate, intermediate and distal; proximate changes could include changes in staff attitudes, values, knowledge and competencies, intermediate could include a sense of workplace coherence as well as changes in organisational resources and practices, and distal could include increased efficacy beliefs, health improvements, patient satisfaction and changes in team climate. Focus group discussions and surveys are among the means by which these domains can be evaluated (Fridrich et al, 2015).

Evaluating effects of the intervention on prescribing:
When learning outcomes from audit activity have been disseminated and implemented, re-auditing is needed to see if recommended changes have occurred, if quality of care has improved, and to close the audit loop (Potter et al, 2010, Tidy and Harding, 2014, BCPFT 2015). Re-auditing a year after guideline dissemination will be the main evaluation of its effects on prescribing. Retrospective data will be collected for the period following guideline dissemination, and results will again be presented to stakeholders. Where audit findings identify non-compliance, an action plan must be developed to identify what changes are required to improve compliance and current practice (BCPFT 2015).

Effective interventions consider target group attitudes towards the behaviour targeted for change and the economic acceptability of the intervention, and recognise diversity in people's values; changing behaviour may not be a priority for a target group (NICE, 2007). Johnston et al (2000) found that 68% of junior staff altered their practice following audit, although consultants were more sceptical. In the Nazareth et al (2002) study, despite GPs' satisfaction with pharmacists' outreach visits and their knowledge of guidelines, there was only a 'modest' effect on prescribing practice. The main barriers found were organisational difficulties, GPs' scepticism, and lack of interest in changing prescribing behaviour.

Evaluating clinical effectiveness:
RCTs are the 'gold standard' for establishing the effectiveness of interventions (Sackett, 1996, Moore et al, 2015). This step has already been taken in the studies on which the six systematic reviews are based. In this small-scale project, an RCT would not be feasible for reasons of cost and delay, and

there are already recent relevant systematic reviews available (Maher et al, 2011, Craig et al, 2012, Spielmans et al, 2013, Veale et al, 2014).

Patient-reported outcome measures or PROMs (Greenhalgh 2014, Thornicroft and Slade, 2014) can be completed by patients or by others on their behalf. Researchers determine which subjective outcomes they wish to measure in patient surveys, for example reduction in psychiatric symptoms, medication side-effects, and so on. The major psychiatric disorders discussed in this project have self-rated questionnaires available, such as the Beck Depression Inventory and Patient Health Questionnaire, both for depression. HONOS, the Health of the Nation Outcome Scale, is used in my trust, and widely in the UK and other Western countries (Thornicroft and Slade, 2014). It includes staff-rated questions on social and physical difficulties of patients, as well as psychopathology. Improved scores in such questionnaires can be used as part of evaluating clinical effectiveness following interventions.

Concluding the evaluation and intervention sustainability:

For the full-scale audit, assistance with data analysis will need to be sought from the trust's clinical audit department; statistical analysis may be involved (Potter et al, 2010). Analysis of quantitative process data usually involves descriptive statistics relating to questions such as fidelity, dose and reach (Moore et al, 2015). After the evaluation has been concluded, a written report will need to be produced and submitted to the Clinical Effectiveness office, and feedback on the evaluation's findings and any actions required will need to be provided (SNFT 2015). Detailed accounts of interventions and standard reports of evaluation methods and findings enable replication studies or wider-scale implementation (Craig et al, 2008).

Long-term sustainability of the intervention will require consideration (Datta and Petticrew, 2013). Behaviour change interventions can effectively modify behaviour, but behaviour change maintenance is rarely maintained, and intervention effects diminish over time (Kwasnicka et al 2016). Ongoing evaluation in the form of periodic re-audits, repeat presentations and re-issues, will encourage future compliance with the guideline, and ongoing monitoring will help to detect adverse events or long-term outcomes unobserved in the original evaluation (Craig et al, 2008). Over time the guideline will need updating in line with emerging research.

Chapter 6: Conclusion

This project had as its initial aim to find out the common non-psychotic psychiatric disorders in which SGAs had been found effective. These have been identified as depression, generalised anxiety disorder, obsessive-compulsive disorder, post-traumatic stress disorder and emotionally unstable personality disorder. However, the usefulness of SGAs may sometimes be limited by their tolerability (Cowen et al 2012). Although associated with fewer neurological side-effects than first-generation antipsychotics, SGAs have been found to be associated with significant physical side-effects such as weight gain (Leucht et al, 2009), diabetes (Kendall 2011, Ipser and Stein 2014), cardiac arrhythmias (Cowen et al 2012), hyperprolactinaemia and hyperlipidaemia (Stoffers et al 2010).

They are also expensive, and their cost-effectiveness has not been conclusively proved (Leucht et al, 2009, Kendall, 2011). There is world-wide concern around the increasing costs of psychotropic medications, which Ilyas and Moncrieff (2012) suggest could be partly due to the requirement for longer-term treatment as well as population growth. They recommend that in order to reduce costs and ensure appropriate and effective use of these medications, further research into prescription patterns is needed to identify more accurately the indications for which these medications are used, particularly off-label.

It has been suggested that some pharmaceutical companies tend to release data exaggerating positive findings on SGA safety and efficacy, and downplaying the negative. Spielman and Parry (2010) recommend changes in dissemination of information on pharmaceutical trials, with better public access to raw data instead of selectively-reported outcomes. This would allow the validity of trial results to be more accurately assessed, meaning that the safest, most effective treatment was delivered to patients.

Influencing clinicians to change prescribing habits depends on complex interactions between many factors, including quality of evidence, confidence and resourcefulness of trainers, characteristics of target group, and context. Knowledge does not necessarily translate into action, as a result of organisational and other barriers (Nazareth et al, 2002).

Considering the prolonged periods over which many psychiatric patients receive psychotropic medications (Ilyas and Moncrieff 2012), often years rather than months, there must always be a careful risk-benefit assessment by clinicians when antipsychotics are prescribed for non-psychotic disorders. More research into long-term effects of atypical antipsychotics is also required, relating to both therapeutic effects and adverse side-effects. There is a need for larger placebo-controlled trials (Ipser and Stein 2012), longer observation periods in studies, and inclusion in trials of participants with psychiatric comorbidities, making findings more generalizable to "real-life" patients (Stoffers et al 2010).

Given their demonstrated side-effects, before SGAs are considered for non-psychotic disorders, other recommended interventions should first have been tried. There may well be a case for avoiding antipsychotics in non-psychotic disorders, except where distress or disruption to a patient's life make the health risks worth taking. Alexander et al (2011) recommend that further 'expansion' of SGA use should be approached cautiously, while awaiting new evidence of their comparative benefits.

References

1. Alexander, G. C., Gallagher, S. A., Mascola, A., Moloney, R. M., Stafford, R. S. (2011) Increasing off-label use of antipsychotic medications in the United States, 1995–2008. *Pharmacoepidemiology and Drug Safety*, 20(2), pp. 177-184.

2. Aveyard, H., Sharp, P. (2013) *A Beginner's Guide to Evidence-based Practice in Health and Social Care*. Berkshire: McGraw-Hill Education.

3. Bandura, A., Walters, R. H. (1977) Social learning theory. New York: General Learning Press.

4. Beach, J., Oates, J. (2014) Information governance and record keeping in community practice. *Community Practitioner*, 87(2), pp. 43-47.

5. Benjamin, A. (2008) Audit: how to do it in practice. *British Medical Journal*, 336 (7655), pp.1241-1245.

6. Benson, N. (2007) *Introducing Psychology: a graphic guide*. Cambridge: Icon Books Ltd.

7. Biggam, J. (2015) *Succeeding with your Master's Dissertation: A Step-by-Step Handbook*. 3rd edition. McGraw-Hill Education (UK).

8. Black Country Partnership NHS Foundation Trust (2015) *Clinical Audit Policy*. West Bromwich: BCPFT.

9. Caldicott, F. (2013). *Information: To share or not to share. The Information Governance Review*. London: Department of Health.

10. Cameron, M., Cranfield, S., Iles, V. (2001) *Making informed decisions on change*. London: London School of Hygiene.

11. Campbell, N. C., Murray, E., Darbyshire, J., et al (2007) Designing and evaluating complex interventions to improve health care. *British Medical Journal*, 334(7591), pp. 455-459.

12. Cane, J., O'Connor, D., & Michie, S. (2012) Validation of the theoretical domains framework for use in behaviour change and implementation research. *Implementation Science*, 7(1), pp.1.

13. Cowen, P., Harrison, P., Burns, T. (2012) *Shorter Oxford Textbook of Psychiatry*. 6th ed. Oxford: Oxford University Press.

14. Craig, P., Dieppe, P., Macintyre, et al (2008) for the Medical Research Council. *Developing and Evaluating Complex Interventions: New Guidance*. London: Medical Research Council.

15. Craig, P., Dieppe, P., Macintyre, S. et al (2012) Developing and evaluating complex interventions: The new Medical Research Council guidance. International Journal of Nursing Studies, 50, pp. 587-592.

16. *Critical Appraisal Skills Programme (CASP) 2013. CASP Checklists Oxford. CASP. Available at:* http://media.wix.com/ugd/dded87_a02ff2e3445f4952992d5a96ca562576.pdf

17. Crowe, M., Sheppard, L. (2011) A review of critical appraisal tools show they lack rigor: alternative tool structure is proposed. *Journal of Clinical Epidemiology*, 64(1), pp. 79-89.

18. Crystal, S., Olfson, M., Huang, C., et al (2009) Broadened use of atypical antipsychotics: safety, effectiveness, and policy challenges. *Health Affairs*, 28(5), w770-w781.

19. Darzi, A. (2008) *High quality care for all: NHS next stage review final report* (Vol. 7432). London: The Stationery Office.

20. Datta, J., Petticrew, M. (2013) Challenges to evaluating complex interventions: a content analysis of published papers. *BioMed Central Public Health*, 13(568), pp.1-18.

21. Department of Health, Self Governing Hospitals (1989) *Working for patients*. London, Department of Health.

22. Department of Health (2003) *Strengthening accountability; involving patients and the public*. London: Department of Health.

23. Depping, A. M., Komossa, K., Kissling, W., Leucht, S. (2010) Second-generation antipsychotics for anxiety disorders. *Cochrane Database of Systematic Reviews 2010*(12), doi:10.1002/14651858.CD008120.pub2.

24. Donabedian, A. (1988) The quality of care: how can it be assessed? *Journal of the American Medical Association*, 260(12), pp. 1743-1748.

25. Fawkes, C. (2000) *A brief introduction to clinical audit*. London: Clinical Audit Central Office.

26. Fineout-Overholt, E., Johnston, L. (2005) Teaching EBP: Asking searchable, answerable clinical questions. *Worldviews on Evidence-Based Nursing*, 2(3), pp. 57-160.

27. Fineout-Overholt, E., O'Mathúna, D. P., Kent, B. (2008) How systematic reviews can foster evidence-based clinical decisions. *Worldviews on Evidence-Based Nursing*, 5(1), pp. 45-48.

28. Fineout-Overholt, E., Williamson, K. M., Gallagher-Ford, L., Melnyk, B. M., Stillwell, S. B. (2011) Evidence-based practice, step by step: following the evidence: planning for sustainable change. *The American Journal of Nursing*, 111(1), pp. 54-60.

29. Francis, J. J., Stockton, C., Eccles, M. P., et al (2009) Evidence-based selection of theories for designing behaviour change interventions: Using methods based on theoretical construct domains to understand clinicians' blood transfusion behaviour. *British Journal of Health Psychology*, 14(4), pp. 625-646.

30. Fridrich, A., Jenny, G. J., Bauer, G. F. (2015) The context, process, and outcome evaluation model for organisational health interventions. *BioMed Research International, 2015*. Accessed: 24/10/16.
    Available at: https://www.hindawi.com/journals/bmri/2015/414832/abs/

31. Gallagher-Ford, L., Fineout-Overholt, E., Melnyk, B. M., & Stillwell, S. B. (2011) Evidence-Based Practice, Step by Step: Rolling Out the Rapid Response Team. *The American Journal of Nursing*, 111(5), pp. 42-47.

32. Greenhalgh, T. (2014) *How to read a paper: The basics of evidence-based medicine*. 5th ed. Oxford: Wiley-Blackwell.

33. Hardman, E., Joughlin, C. (1998) *Focus on Clinical Audit in Child and Adolescent Mental Health Services*. London: The Royal College of Psychiatrists.

34. Haw, C., Stubbs, J. (2007) Off-label use of antipsychotics: are we mad? *Expert Opinion on Drug Safety* 6(5), pp. 533-545.

35. Hogg, C. N. (2007) Patient and public involvement: what next for the NHS? *Health Expectations*, 10(2), pp. 129-138.

36. Ilyas, S., Moncrieff, J. (2012) Trends in prescriptions and costs of drugs for mental disorders in England, 1998–2010. *The British Journal of Psychiatry*, 200(5), pp. 393-398.

37. Ipser, J. C., Stein, D. J. (2012) Evidence-based pharmacotherapy of post-traumatic stress disorder (PTSD). *The International Journal of Neuropsychopharmacology*, 15(06), pp. 825-840.

38. Johnston, G., Crombie, I. K., Alder, E. M., Davies, H. T. O., Millard, A. (2000) Reviewing audit: barriers and facilitating factors for effective clinical audit. *Quality in Health Care*, *9*(1), pp.23-36.

39. Kendall, T. (2011) The rise and fall of the atypical antipsychotics. *The British Journal of Psychiatry*, 199(4), pp. 266-268.

40. Kwasnicka, D., Dombrowski, S. U., White, M., Sniehotta, F. (2016) Theoretical explanations for maintenance of behaviour change: a systematic review of behaviour theories. *Health Psychology Review*, pp. 1-20.

41. Leucht, S., Corves, C., Arbter, D., Engel, R. R., Li, C., Davis, J. M. (2009) Second-generation versus first-generation antipsychotic drugs for schizophrenia: a meta-analysis. *The Lancet*, *373*(9657), pp. 31-41.

42. Maher, A. R., Maglione, M., Bagley, et al (2011) Efficacy and comparative effectiveness of atypical antipsychotic medications for off-label uses in adults: a systematic review and meta-analysis. *Journal of the American Medical Association*, 306(12), pp.1359-1369.

43. Marston, L., Nazareth, I., Petersen, I., Walters, K., Osborn, D. P. (2014) Prescribing of antipsychotics in UK primary care: a cohort study. *British Medical Journal Open*, 4(12), e006135.

44. McKean, A., Monasterio, E. (2014) Indications of atypical antipsychotics in the elderly. *Expert Review of Clinical Pharmacology*, *8*(1), pp. 5-7.

45. Melnyk, B. M., Fineout-Overholt, E. (2005) Rapid critical appraisal of randomized controlled trials (RCTs): an essential skill for evidence-based practice (EBP). *Pediatric Nursing*, 31(1), pp. 50-52.

46. Melnyk, B. M., Fineout-Overholt, E., Stillwell, S. B., Williamson, K. M. (2010) Evidence-based practice: step by step: the seven steps of evidence-based practice. *The American Journal of Nursing*, 110(1), pp. 51-53.

47. Melnyk, B. M., Fineout-Overholt, E., Gallagher-Ford, L., Stillwell, S. B. (2011) Evidence-based practice, step by step: sustaining evidence-based practice through organizational policies and an innovative model. *The American Journal of Nursing*, 111(9), pp. 57-60.

48. Moore, G. F., Audrey, S., Barker, M., et al (2015) Process evaluation of complex interventions: Medical Research Council guidance. B*ritish Medical Journal*, *350*, h1258.

49. National Institute for Clinical Excellence (2002) *Principles for best practice in clinical audit.* Oxford: Radcliffe Publishing.

50. National Institute for Health and Clinical Excellence (2005a) *Post-traumatic stress disorder: management.* NICE clinical guideline CG26.

51. National Institute for Health and Clinical Excellence (2005b) *Obsessive-compulsive disorder and body dysmorphic disorder: treatment.* NICE clinical guideline CG31.

52. National Institute for Health and Care Excellence (2007) Behaviour change; general approaches. NICE clinical guideline PH6.

53. National Institute for Health and Clinical Excellence (2009) *Borderline personality disorder: recognition and management.* NICE clinical guideline CG78.

54. National Institute for Health and Clinical Excellence (2011) *Generalised anxiety disorder and panic disorder in adults: management.* NICE clinical guideline CG 113.

55. National Institute for Health and Clinical Excellence (2012) *The treatment and management of depression in adults* (update). NICE clinical guideline CG90.

56. National Institute for Health and Clinical Excellence (2015) *Personality disorders; borderline and antisocial.* NICE quality standard QS88.

57. Nazareth, I., Freemantle, N., Duggan, et al (2002) Evaluation of a complex intervention for changing professional behaviour: the Evidence Based Out Reach (EBOR) Trial. *Journal of Health Services Research and Policy,* 7(4), pp. 230-238.

58. Palmer, C. (2002) Clinical governance: breathing new life into clinical audit. *Advances in Psychiatric Treatment,* 8(6), pp. 470-476.

59. Potter, J., Fuller, C., Ferris, M. (2010) Local clinical audit: handbook for physicians. London: Healthcare Quality Improvement Partnership.

60. Provenzale, J. M., Stanley, R. J. (2006) A systematic guide to reviewing a manuscript. *Journal of Nuclear Medicine Technology,* 34(2), pp. 92-99.

61. Renedo, A., Marston, C. A., Spyridonidis, D., Barlow, J. (2015) Patient and public involvement in healthcare quality improvement: How organizations can help patients and professionals to collaborate. *Public Management Review,* 17(1), pp. 17-34.

62. Sackett, D. L., Rosenberg, W. M., Gray, J. M., Haynes, R. B., Richardson, W. S. (1996) Evidence based medicine: what it is and what it isn't. *British Medical Journal,* 312(7023), pp. 71-72.

63. Sadler-Moore, D. (2010) Evidence-based Practice Project Module. *Della Analysis of a research article GRID 2010.*
Available at:
https://wolf.wlv.ac.uk/iohp/81444/Della%20Analysis%20of%20a%20research%20article%20GRID%202010.doc?menu=1532546

64. Salisbury NHS Foundation Trust (2015) *Service Evaluation Guidance.* Salisbury: Salisbury NHS Foundation Trust.

65. Semple, D., Smyth, R. (2013) *Oxford Handbook of Psychiatry.* Oxford: Oxford University Press.

66. Spielmans, G. I., Parry, P. I. (2010) From evidence-based medicine to marketing-based medicine: evidence from internal industry documents. *Journal of Bioethical Inquiry,* 7(1), pp.13-29.

67. Spielmans, G. I., Berman, M. I., Linardatos, E., Rosenlicht, N. Z., Perry, A., Tsai, A. C. (2013) Adjunctive atypical antipsychotic treatment for major depressive disorder: a meta-analysis of depression, quality of life, and safety outcomes. *PLOS Medicine*, *10*(3), e1001403.

68. Stoffers, J., Völlm, B. A., Rücker, G., Timmer, A., Huband, N., Lieb, K. (2010) Pharmacological interventions for borderline personality disorder. *The Cochrane Database of Systematic Reviews*, 16 (6), CD005653.

69. The British House of Parliament (1998) *The Data Protection Act*. London: the Stationery Office. Accessed 24/10/16. Available at: http://www.legislation.gov.uk/ukpga/1998/29/contents

70. Thornicroft, G., Slade, M. (2014) New trends in assessing the outcomes of mental health interventions. *World Psychiatry*, *13*(2), pp.118-124.

71. Tidy, C., Harding, M. (2014) Audit and audit cycle. *Patient*. Accessed 31/10/16. Available at: http://patient.info/doctor/audit-and-audit-cycle/

72. Veale, D. M., Miles, S. K., Smallcombe, et al (2014) Atypical antipsychotic augmentation in SSRI treatment refractory obsessive-compulsive disorder: a systematic review and meta-analysis. *BMC Psychiatry*, 14(1), pp. 317.

73. Wallace, J. (2011) The practice of evidence-based psychiatry today. *Advances in Psychiatric Treatment*, 17(5), pp. 389-395.

74. World Health Organisation (1992) *The ICD-10 Classification of Mental and Behavioural Disorders: Clinical Descriptions and Diagnostic Guidelines*. Geneva: WHO.

Appendix 1

Sadler-Moore deconstruction grid completed for Maher et al (2011) study

TOPIC: Analysis of a Published Research Article Della Sadler-Moore **A grid to aid you to identify the stages of the research process reported in your research article prior to performing a critical review of the research.**	

AREA TO REVIEW	YOUR FINDINGS
What is the title of the chosen research article?	'Efficacy and comparative effectiveness of atypical antipsychotic medications for off-label uses in adults.'
What are the aims of the research eg the study question(s), hypothesis, problem statement etc	To perform a systematic review on the efficacy and safety of atypical antipsychotic medications for use in conditions lacking approval for labelling and marketing by the US Food and Drug Administration.
Who is the researcher(s), and what are his / her relationship to the study? eg qualifications, reason given for conducting the study.	Maher et al (2011) 4 researchers M.D.s., one also PhD. Others MPP or MS. Dr. Maher was affiliated to Southern California Evidence-based Practice Centre.
What is the context / background / rationale for conducting a study of this nature.	The use of atypical antipsychotic medications is rapidly increasing in the United States. The estimated use of these drugs for off-label indications, meaning those without FDA approval for these indications, doubled between 1995 and 2008. (At the time of the report, atypicals were approved for the treatment of schizophrenia, bipolar disorder and depression, but were, and are, commonly used as well for such conditions as agitation in dementia, anxiety and obsessive-compulsive disorder).
The literature review: is there a review of the literature, how does this relate to the study? eg theoretical literature, policy literature, empirical literature.	No formal literature review, but studies and articles were referenced through the various sections of the report.
The Research Design. What type of research is reported, e.g. survey, experiment, ethnography etc.	Quantitative; systematic review of randomised controlled trials.
The population, Sample and Sampling Method:	Patients prescribed atypical antipsychotic medications for off-label indications.

How would you describe the type of research data that was collected eg words, numbers etc	Numerical.
What Method(s) / techniques were used to collect the research data e.g. Questionnaire Interview Schedule Physiological measurements Observation	Searches of PubMed, EMBASE, CINAHL, PsycInfo, Cochrane DARE, and CENTRAL through May 2011 for studies of atypical antipsychotic medications including aripiprazole, asenapine, iloperidone, olanzapine, paliperidone, quetiapine, risperidone, and ziprasidone. Clozapine was excluded due to its almost exclusive use for schizophrenia. Search terms included the drug names and terms for the conditions previously described. They included depression for drugs without FDA approval for this indication. Regulatory documents from the FDA and Health Canada were searched. They performed reference mining of relevant reviews. They included only studies published in the English language. Clinical trials were used to assess efficacy outcomes. Adverse events were abstracted from clinical trials and large observational studies.
Was a Pilot Study conducted ? if so what was the justification for this and what were the outcomes of conducting it. Eg How many included, findings, any modifications	No.
By what specific approaches were the data collection methods used with the sample e.g. postal, telephone, personal, trained others (+ if applicable what were the response rates).	Trained investigators. Relevant outcomes were selected by trained psychiatrists. 4 investigators independently reviewed titles and abstracts for potentially relevant articles. They abstracted data from full-text articles using structured review forms, and disagreements were resolved by consensus. Statisticians abstracted outcome data (verified by a clinician-investigator) for the pooled analysis. One investigator abstracted data on adverse events, and these were checked by a second reviewer.
What techniques were used to manage the research data that had been collected. eg transcribing, computer package usage, data analysis frameworks...	Computer package usage(meta-analyses conducted using Stata statistical software version 10.0 and StatXact procs version 9) Internal validity, quality of clinical trials, internal validity of observational studies, effect sizes, strength of evidence and bias were assessed.
How were the research findings reported? eg thematically, narratives, tables, pie charts, verbatim quotations	Narratives and tables.

What were the major research findings? How do they relate to the aims of the study?	Evidence was demonstrated only for a few of the off-label conditions being treated with SGAs.
	Quetiapine showed significant benefit in generalised anxiety disorder, and risperidone in OCD. Aripiprazole, olanzapine and risperidone showed small benefit for behavioural symptoms in dementia, but but adverse events were likely with olanzapine and risperidone, and there was an increase in risk of strokes and death in the elderly.
	Evidence did not support the use of atypical antipsychotics in substance misuse or eating disorders, and evidence on their use in insomnia was inconclusive.
	Adverse side-effects with atypicals were common.
What ethical issues were acknowledged?	None, as it was secondary research based on previous clinical trials.
What were the researchers conclusions from conducting the study?	Benefits and harms vary among atypical antipsychotic medications for off-label use. Adverse effects are common. Other conclusions as in research findings above.
What issues of reliability, validity or rigor / trustworthiness were acknowledged in the study.	'Unidentified, unpublished or excluded studies might have reported results different from those included here.
	'Studies published after June 1, 2011, including a recent large randomized controlled trial of risperidone therapy for patients with military-related PTSD and symptoms resistant to SSRIs, were not included in our review.
	'We detected unexplained heterogeneity, which may indicate the presence of publication bias, in our pooled results for OCD. This finding accordingly tempers our conclusion about OCD.
	'Our meta-analysis, particularly for dementia, distills broad heterogeneities across patient and treatment circumstances, and the studies used variable definitions and measures of agitation, which complicates the clinical interpretation and application of the findings. Even so, the evidence is reasonably consistent regarding a small improvement, on average, in clinically relevant symptoms for patients with dementia.
	'We did not compare atypical antipsychotic medications to nonpharmacological therapy. Sixth, we found no studies on off-label use for the 3 newer atypical antipsychotic medications (asenapine, iloperidone, or paliperidone).
	'Lastly, most studies were sponsored by drug manufacturers (for example, 27 of 38 dementia trials and 12 of 14 anxiety trials). The existence of the CATIE-AD study, which was federally sponsored and reported results consistent with the industry-sponsored studies, increases our confidence in the conclusions regarding atypical antipsychotic medications for elderly patients with dementia.'
Are there any additional issues of note regarding this research study ?	Cardiac QT interval prolongation by atypicals, an important side-effect, did not appear to be emphasised.

Appendix 2

CASP critical appraisal tool used with Maher et al (2011) study

<u>CASP checklist for systematic reviews:</u>	<u>Maher et al 2011</u>
Did the review address a clearly focused question?	Yes, the safety and efficacy of atypical antipsychotics for use in conditions lacking FDA approval.
Did the authors look for the right type of papers?	Yes, RCTs.
Do you think all the important, relevant studies were included?	Only those published in English.
Did the review's authors do enough to assess the quality of the included studies?	Yes.
If the results of the review have been combined, was it reasonable to do so?	Analyses were pooled for trials carried out on individual disorders, and robust measures were taken to assess validity.
What are the overall results of the review?	Evidence was demonstrated only for a few of the off-label conditions being treated with atypicals. Quetiapine showed significant benefit in generalised anxiety disorder, and risperidone in OCD. Aripiprazole, olanzapine and risperidone showed small benefit for behavioural symptoms in dementia, but but adverse events were likely with olanzapine and risperidone, and there was an increase in risk of strokes and death in the elderly. Evidence did not support the use of atypical antipsychotics in substance misuse or eating disorders, and evidence on their use in insomnia was inconclusive. Adverse side-effects with atypicals were common.
How precise are the results? (C.I.)	Variable for different modalities.
Can the results be applied to the local population?	Yes, the psychiatric conditions studied are prevalent in the local population as well.
Were all important outcomes considered?	Relative QTc interval prolongation of the antipsychotics may not have been considered. The relative risks of the individual antipychotics taken in overdose were not considered; this is of particular significance with psychiatric patients.
Are the benefits worth the harms and costs?	In elderly patients with dementia, there was an increased risk of death, so not in their case.

	Risk of metabolic problems and adverse side-effects in patients in general means that risks need to be balanced against benefits, and clinical profiles of each individual patient has to be taken into consideration. In depression unresponsive to antidepressants, the risk may be worth taking if the illness can be life-threatening. If levels of patient distress and interference with functioning are not sufficiently severe with their non-psychotic psychiatric disorder to expose the patient to the potential health risks, especially in the long term, antipsychotics may be better avoided.

Appendix 3

Clinical audit planner
(Based on models by BCFT 2015 and Hardman and Joughlin 1998)

	PROJECT DETAILS
Audit title:	'Atypical antipsychotics in non-psychotic disorders.'
Reason for audit:	To assess current (baseline) prescribing patterns of atypical antipsychotics for non-psychotic disorders in 'CMHT X'
Aims/objectives:	To determine which non-psychotic disorders atypical antipsychotics are currently being prescribed for, and which medications are being used. To encourage evidence-based prescribing of atypical antipsychotics for non-psychotic disorders in the psychiatric service.
Explain how this will benefit patient care:	Ensuring that patients get the most effective medications.
Standards/guidelines:	3. NICE guidelines on treatment of depression, generalised anxiety disorder, obsessive-compulsive disorder, post-traumatic stress disorder and borderline personality disorder. 4. Systematic reviews : Stoffers et al (2010) Depping et al (2011) Maher et al (2011) Ipser and Stein (2012) Spielmans et al (2013) Veale et al (2014).
Audit criteria:	Patients aged between 18 and 65 who attended a psychiatric clinic in 'CMHT X' between January and December 2015, and were prescribed atypical antipsychotics for non-psychotic disorders.
Sample size:	20 patient records fulfilled above audit criteria.
Audit Methodology:	Type: Retrospective Source: Electronic patient records (Care Notes).
Audit tool:	Data collection tool designed.
Patient information to be collected:	Age Sex Ethnicity Diagnosis Atypical antipsychotic prescribed
Clinical lead for project:	Name: Job title:

Proposed project team:	Names: Job titles:
Group:	Mental Health
Service area:	Community
Location	UK
Is this a re-audit?	No.
What professions are involved in this audit?	Medical.
Are any non-trust organisations involved in this audit?	No.
Service user involvement:	Indirect only; data collection is retrospective.
Resources:	Audit tool design, review of patient records and data analysis to be carried out by project lead.
Ethics/confidentiality:	In accordance with Data Protection Act and Caldicott Principles.
Date form completed:	
Proposed report date:	To be arranged.
Reporting arrangements:	Clinicians' forum.
Proposed re-audit date:	1 year following first audit report.

Appendix 4

Data collection tool for baseline audit

Patient Serial no.	Age	Sex	Ethnicity	Primary diagnosis	Any psychiatric comorbidities	Atypical antipsychotic	Use supported by NICE guidelines/systematic review findings?
1							
2							
3							
4							
5							
6							
7							
8							
9							
10							
11							
12							

Completed data collection tool for baseline audit

Patient Serial nos.	Ages	Sex	Ethnicity	Primary diagnosis	Psychiatric comorbidities	SGA(s) over last 1 year	Use supported by NICE guidelines/ systematic review findings?
1		M	British Caucasian	Emotionally unstable personality disorder	Post-traumatic stress disorder	Olanzapine	Improvement of some symptoms in emotionally unstable personality disorder, but increased risk of self-damaging behaviour and metabolic side-effects (Stoffers et al 2010)
2		F	British Caucasian	Emotionally unstable personality disorder	Recurrent depression	Quetiapine	Yes, recommended for depression (NICE 2012, Depping et al 2011, Spilemans et al 2013).
3		F	British Caucasian	Emotionally unstable personality disorder	Mixed anxiety and depression	Risperidone	Recommended for depression (NICE 2012, Spielmans et al 2013).
4		F	British Caucasian	Post-traumatic stress disorder	Recurrent depression	Aripiprazole	Yes, recommended for depression (NICE 2012, Spielmans et al 2013).

5		F	British Caucasian	Emotionally unstable personality disorder		Aripiprazole	Yes (Stoffers et al 2010).
6		M	British Caucasian	Emotionally unstable personality disorder		Quetiapine	Not specifically recommended for this disorder ,and may present overdose risk. However, recommended for depression and effective in anxiety, which are prevalent with this disorder.
7		F	Mixed-race	Emotionally unstable personality disorder	Post-traumatic stress disorder	Aripiprazole	Yes (Stoffers st al 2010).
8		F	British Caucasian	Recurrent depression	Anorexia nervosa	Aripiprazole	Yes (NICE 2012, Spielmans et al (2013).
9		F	British Caucasian	Emotionally unstable personality disorder		Aripiprazole	Yes (Stoffers et al 2010).
10		F	British Caucasian	Emotionally unstable personality disorder		Aripiprazole	Yes (Stoffers et al 2010).
11		M	British Caucasian	Emotionally unstable personality disorder	Post-traumatic stress disorder	Olanzapine	Improvement of some symptoms in emotionally unstable personality disorder, but increased risk of self-damaging behaviour and metabolic side-effects (Stoffers et al 2010) Reduces symptoms in PTSD used as an adjunct to SSRIs, but significant weight gain (Ipser and Stein 2012).
12		F	British Caucasian	Emotionally unstable personality disorder	Unspecified anxiety disorder	Risperidone	Effective for depressive symptoms (NICE 2012, Spielmans et al 2013).

13		F	British Caucasian	Emotionally unstable personality disorder		Aripiprazole	Yes, `effective in emotionally unstable personality disorder (Stoffers et al 2010).
14		M	British Caucasian	Recurrent depression	Generalised anxiety disorder	Quetiapine	Yes (NICE 2012, Depping et al 2011, Spielmans et al 2013).
15		F	Black African	Depression		Aripiprazole	Yes (NICE 2012, Spielmans et al 2013).
16		F	British Caucasian	Emotionally unstable personality disorder		Aripiprazole	Yes (Stoffers et al 2010).
17		F	British Caucasian	Emotionally unstable personality disorder	Mixed anxiety and depression Asperger's syndrome	Risperidone	Effective in depression (NICE 2012, Spielmans et al 2013).
18		F	British Caucasian	Emotionally unstable personality disorder		Risperidone	Helpful with depressive symptoms (NICE 2012, Spielmans et al 2013).
19		F	British Caucasian	Emotionally unstable personality disorder	Opiate dependence Alcohol misuse	Olanzapine	Improvement of some symptoms in emotionally unstable personality disorder, but increased risk of self-damaging behaviour and metabolic side-effects (Stoffers et al 2010). Could also potentiate sedative effects of alcohol and opiates.
20		F	British Caucasian	Recurrent depression	Obsessive-compulsive disorder	Aripiprazole	Yes, recommended for both depression and OCD (NICE 2012, Spielmans et al 2013, Veale et al 2014).

Data collection tool for re-audit

Patient Serial no.	Age	Sex	Ethnicity	Primary diagnosis	Any psychiatric comorbidities	SGA(s) prescribed in last 1 year following issue of guideline	Use supported by NICE guidelines/systematic reviews?
1							
2							
3							
4							
5							
6							
7							
8							
9							
10							
11							
12							

Appendix 5

Draft guideline for the use of atypical antipsychotics in non-psychotic disorders

Psychiatric disorder	Atypical antipsychotic recommended by NICE guidelines?	Atypical antipsychotic found effective by systematic review?
Depression	Only when treatment with antidepressants and psychological interventions have failed or shown inadequate response, consider augmenting with an antipsychotic such as **aripiprazole, olanzapine, quetiapine or risperidone** (NICE 2012).	Depping et al (2011) – significantly better response to **quetiapine** than placebo. Monotherapy with quetiapine appeared to be as efficacious as low-dose SSRIs. Spielmans et al (2013) -statistically significant effects on remission of depression with **aripiprazole, quetiapine, risperidone** and a combination of **olanzapine** with fluoxetine.
Generalised anxiety disorder (GAD)	Antipsychotics should not be offered for GAD in primary care. No specific antipsychotic recommended. (NICE 2011)	Depping et al (2011) - significantly better response to **quetiapine** in GAD than placebo. However, not officially registered for treating GAD. Maher et al (2011) - significant benefit in GAD with **quetiapine.** Depping et al (2011) - **Olanzapine** added to antidepressants significantly reduced anxiety, but produced significantly more sedation and weight gain.
Emotionally unstable personality disorder	Antipsychotics can be used to treat transient psychotic symptoms. Not for medium to long-term treatment, and not for the individual symptoms/behaviour associated with emotionally unstable personality disorder. (NICE 2009) NICE (2015) quality standards indicate that patients can be prescribed antipsychotic or sedative medication only for short-term crisis management or treatment of comorbid conditions.	Stoffers et al (2010) - significant effects with **aripiprazole** in reduction of impulsivity, anger, depression, paranoid symptoms and anxiety associated with the disorder. Also less likely to engage in self-mutilation. With **olanzapine** significant reductions in affective instability, anger, paranoia and anxiety associated with the disorder. However, self-damaging behaviour more likely, and metabolic side-effects are significant.

Post-traumatic stress disorder (PTSD)	**Olanzapine** can be used as an adjunct to antidepressants and psychological interventions if condition is resistant. (NICE 2005a)	Maher et al (2011) - moderate evidence of benefit for **risperidone** in PTSD. Ipser and Stein (2012) – significant reduction of symptom severity with adjunctive **risperidone** in PTSD found. **Olanzapine** also found to significantly reduce symptom severity used as an adjunct to SSRIs. Significant weight gain with olanzapine.
Obsessive-compulsive disorder (OCD)	Antipsychotics can be used as adjuncts if condition is resistant to antidepressants and psychological interventions. Not for use as monotherapy. No specific antipsychotic identified. (NICE 2005b)	Maher et al (2011) - significant benefit from **risperidone** in OCD. Veale et al (2014) - limited evidence of low dose **risperidone** and **aripiprazole** in the short term.
Panic disorder	Antipsychotics should not be prescribed. (NICE 2011)	Depping et al (2011) - No trials identified.